EARLY MEDIEVAL MEDICINE

EARLY MEDIEVAL MEDICINE

WITH SPECIAL REFERENCE TO FRANCE
AND CHARTRES

LOREN C. MacKINNEY

ARNO PRESS
A New York Times Company
New York • 1979

Editorial Supervision: Mary Kay Hamalainen

Reprint Edition 1979 by Arno Press Inc.

JOHNS HOPKINS UNIVERSITY PRESS REPRINTS
ISBN for complete set: 0-405-10575-4
See last pages of this volume for titles.

Manufactured in the United States of America

Library of Congress Cataloging in Publication Data

MacKinney, Loren Carey, 1891-
    Early medieval medicine.

    (Johns Hopkins University Press reprints)
    Reprint of the ed. published by Johns Hopkins
Press, Baltimore, which was issued as v. 3 of the
Publications of the Institute of the History of
Medicine, Johns Hopkins University, 3d ser., The
Hideyo Noguchi lectures.
    Bibliography: p.
    1. Medicine, Medieval. 2. Medicine--France--
History. 3. Medicine--France--Chartres--History.
I. Title. II. Series: Johns Hopkins University.
Institute of the History of Medicine. Publications.
3d ser., The Hideyo Noguchi lectures ; v. 3.
[DNLM: WZ54 M158e 1937a]
R141.M3 1979   610'.944   78-19254
ISBN 0-405-10613-0

EARLY MEDIEVAL MEDICINE:

WITH SPECIAL REFERENCE TO FRANCE AND CHARTRES

PUBLICATIONS OF THE INSTITUTE OF THE HISTORY
OF MEDICINE

THE JOHNS HOPKINS UNIVERSITY

LONDON: HUMPHREY MILFORD
OXFORD UNIVERSITY PRESS

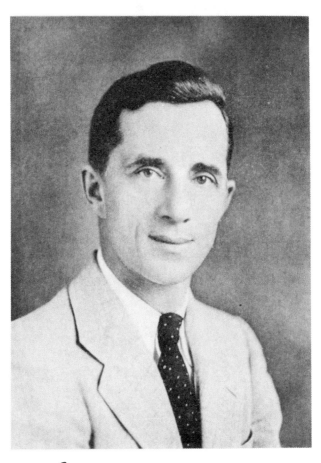

Loren C. MacKinney

PUBLICATIONS OF THE INSTITUTE OF THE HISTORY OF MEDICINE
THE JOHNS HOPKINS UNIVERSITY
THIRD SERIES   VOLUME III

EARLY MEDIEVAL MEDICINE

WITH SPECIAL REFERENCE TO FRANCE
AND CHARTRES

BY

LOREN C. MacKINNEY, PH. D.
Professor of Medieval History
University of North Carolina

THE HIDEYO NOGUCHI LECTURES

BALTIMORE
THE JOHNS HOPKINS PRESS
1937

PRINTED IN THE UNITED STATES OF AMERICA
BY J. H. FURST COMPANY. BALTIMORE, MARYLAND

TABLE OF CONTENTS

I

THE DARK AGE CONCEPT AND EARLY
MEDIEVAL MEDICINE *

THREE years ago on the occasion of the Noguchi Lectures Dr. Castiglioni of the University of Padua paid tribute to one of the most inspiring eras of human progress, presenting in spirited and picturesque language a rich store of information concerning *The Renaissance of Medicine in Italy*. Two years ago, Dr. Zilboorg presented a wealth of interesting evidence concerning *The Medical Man and the Witch during the Renaissance*. I am to direct your attention to a region and period that is perhaps at the opposite extreme of human achievement. Italy during the age of the renascence and France during the so-called " dark age " present as striking a contrast as can be found in medieval history.

* I take this opportunity of expressing my appreciation to the American Council of Learned Societies for a grant in aid, and to the University of North Carolina for a Kenan leave, which made it possible to complete my study of medical manuscripts in a number of European Libraries; also to Dr. J. B. Bullitt and Professors C. W. Beeson, B. L. Ullmann, Elias Lowe, Lynn Thorndike, Frederick M. Carey, Richard H. Shryock, U. T. Holmes, R. W. Linker, Augusto Beccaria, and Dr. Ernest Wickersheimer, for helpful suggestions.

doctors & historians

It is with deliberate intent that I lead your thoughts into a very dim, rather dreary and little understood epoch. Those who have feasted long on the rich fare of the renascence may find little in the earlier middle ages to tempt the mental appetite. But there is in the subject much food for thought, and intensive thought. Such may be as beneficial as it is distasteful at first sight. There is an increasing tendency among modern historians to find worthwhile results in the less popular periods of history.

However much my topic may be lacking in glamor, there is one respect in which I take my place alongside Dr. Castiglioni, Dr. Zilboorg, and others of the modern school of medical historians. This can best be explained by quoting from the editor's introduction to the printed edition of Dr. Castiglioni's lectures. These words were written by the head of this Institute. He stated therein that he, along with the lecturer, held to the belief that " the history of medicine is but one aspect of the history of civilization; that it therefore cannot be studied separately, but has to be traced within the wide range of general culture." [1] These words were more than a polite expression of agreement with a guest speaker. They were the permanent ideal of this Institute and its leader. Within the last year he has penned the following: " The history of medicine is not only medicine, but obviously also history. It is one aspect of the history of civilization." [2]

I trust that I am not presuming when I suggest that it is due to this broad viewpoint that I am honored with the privilege of giving the Noguchi lectures. Never before have they been given by one untrained in the medical profession. The fact that a doctor of philosophy rather than medicine, a professor of medieval rather than medical history has been invited to deliver the 1936 series, indicates a steadfast and, we hope, not unjustified faith in this ideal.

The ideal and its practical application in bringing to this institute lay as well as medical historians, marks an advanced step in American medicine and history. A close rapprochement has long been needed. In an age such as ours, cooperation and exchange of ideas is a necessary antidote against the ignorance of narrow specialization. In this respect it must be admitted that the medical profession has shown more venturesomeness than the historians. Doctors have not hesitated to delve into history. In the past, the writing of medical history has been practically monopolized by physicians, and they have done much to popularize the subject. But this has had its disadvantages, for great physicians do not always write accurate history. So far as historians are concerned there has been too little inclination to invade the realm of medicine. The reason is obvious. It is more difficult for an historian to learn medicine, than for a doctor to learn history. Even though historians have long been of the opinion that their field of study comprises human life in all its aspects, they have hesitated to delve into the history of a specialized science. But medical history can and should be a common ground for the two professions. We trust that the activity of both M. D. and Ph. D. historians in medical history will increase and that it will be profitable to both professions.

As a lay historian I feel that I can contribute more to your knowledge of history than of medicine. Therefore, it is my purpose to emphasize the non-technical aspects of medical practice in the early centuries and to interpret its development as an integral part of the beginnings of modern western civilization.

As an introduction to our survey of medieval medicine, I wish to summarize a few of the historical generalizations that have been, and are still current concerning this era. It is popularly known as the dark age, and I begin with the dark age concept as held by the historical profession.

We dismiss with only a brief comment, the completely discredited idea that the ten centuries from 476 when the Western Empire fell, to 1453 when Constantinople was captured by the Turks, were a dreary abyss of darkness, ignorance and superstition. Today no scholar of any historical reputation clings to this lingering superstition of early modern times. The viewpoint of up to date scholarship has been cogently summarized by a recent commentator.

Dark ages [he writes] is a term formerly used to cover the whole period from the end of the classical civilization to the fifteenth century revival of learning. . . . With the progress of medieval studies in the nineteenth century, it became impossible for historians to dismiss one of the great constructive periods of human activity with such an epithet, and the phrase has now become obsolete.[8]

It is perhaps an exaggeration to assert that the phrase dark age has now become obsolete, but certainly the older use of the term is obsolete. Not even in the high school text books of recent date can one find the title dark age applied to the entire medieval period. About all that remains in undisputed dark-

the dark ages ?
renaissances

ness, is the period from 500 to 1000 A. D., and there are those who question the accuracy of the title for even these centuries.

Without debating this question, one may still ask the *reason* for such a change in historical nomenclature. The answer seems to be that given above; namely the progress of medieval studies. Just as chemists have found valuable by-products in slag and refuse heaps of mines or smelters, so also careful historians have discovered worthwhile material in centuries once considered worthless. For over a century, ever since scholars began to examine the middle ages with serious and sympathetic interest, the period of actual darkness has tended to recede. The earlier as well as the later centuries have caught the attention of seekers for light. And the search has not been fruitless. The recent revaluation of the so-called dark age, with which we are concerned in this lecture, is merely a continuation of the process by which the *later* medieval centuries were moved from darkness into light. The nineteenth century change of scholarly attitude toward the *later* middle ages has a twentieth century sequel which at times threatens to wipe out the dark, or early middle age as a distinct historical epoch.

The term dark age is by no means obsolete, but it is losing much of its sinister reputation. For instance, one of the most recent and most highly praised of all American text books of medieval history contains a chapter with the engaging title " Light in the Dark Ages." [4]

Bit by bit the period of actual darkness in medieval history tends to shrink. If one were not aware of the objective manner in which most medievalists work, it might be suspected that there had been a premeditated campaign for the gradual abolition of the dark age. It might appear as though groups of sappers and miners, beginning at both ends of the middle ages, had slowly driven the dark age from one line of entrenchments to another. For example, years ago it was discovered that renascence characteristics existed centuries before Petrarch and his humanist followers. In place of the opinion that there was nothing but cultural darkness before the fourteenth century, it was recognized that the thirteenth century made remarkable progress,[5] and that there was a twelfth century renascence.[6] French scholars now make constant reference to an eleventh century " renaissance "; in fact they push its beginnings back to the middle or end of the tenth century.[7] This, it will be noted, brings the end of the dark age to within about one hundred years of the Carolingian renascence of the ninth century. But even in the brief intervening period the defenders of the dark age tradition are harassed by references to an Ottonian renascence in the Rhinelands at about 950, and to Alfred's remarkable achievements a half century earlier in raising the status of civilization in England. As a consequence the tenth century, which once vied with the seventh century for the reputation of being " the most ignorant, the darkest and the most barbarous period ever seen," [8] threatens to become a renascence outpost.

It is obvious that the ninth, tenth, and eleventh centuries are tending to desert the dark age and join the renascence forces. I say " tending," because even the most optimistic of historians recognize that in all regions during these centuries there was disorder and barbarism. But it is coming to be generally recognized that the centuries following the reign of Charles the Great saw continuous progress in civilization, even amid the occasional ravages of Norse, Moslem, and Hungarian invaders. [9]

At the other end of the dark age, also, in the history of the period before the Carolingian renascence, the indefatigable efforts of patient researchers have unearthed evidence that forces somewhat of a revaluation. For instance, after 476, the traditional date at which " the light of culture was snuffed out " in the West, there is indisputable evidence of civilized life. Theodoric, the Ostrogothic ruler of Italy from 493 to 526, instituted a veritable renascence of Roman economic and cultural life. A century later, in barbarian controlled regions of the West, there were so many eminent scholars that the year 600 A. D. might with some justification be made the focal point for another early medieval renascence.

The 200 years between this epoch and the age of Charles the Great are of darker hue. There were, however, Irishmen of high intellectual attainments in many continental monasteries, and England, at about 700, produced the incomparable Bede. And so as one reviews the results of research on the middle ages, it seems at first glance that very little of actual darkness remains.

Such conclusions might be accepted unconditionally if one relied on the most optimistic reports. For instance, a writer on the history of literature expresses the following opinion;

We used to talk of the Dark Ages; most of us know by

now that the true Dark Ages came before the true Middle Ages; and that in many ways the Middle Ages were far from dark. But, following the figure of an age of darkness, we are apt to think of [it as] an age of twilight; or perhaps of grey morning light. . . . It would be truer to compare even the Dark Ages to a dark room, with certain chinks in the shutters through which particular rays of light could pierce. But the light was daylight, what there was of it; and not even a dull or troubled daylight. It was broad daylight that came through a narrow hole. Or it was like some long narrow ray of a searchlight sent out from a great city and falling like a spotlight on a remote village or a lonely man. And just as any man, however much in darkness, if he looks right down the searchlight, looks into a furnace of white-hot radiance, so any medieval man who had the luck to hear the right lectures or look at the right manuscript, did not merely ' follow a gleam,' a grey glimmer in a mystical forest; but looked straight down the ages into the adiant mind of Aristotle. . . .[10]

In direct contrast, however, another writer viewing the same period paints the following gloomy picture:

Although the Graeco-Roman world did not sink under a catastrophic blow such as wiped out Babylon and Susa etc. . . . although its downfall was a process of transitional, though rapid, disintegration rather than a sudden and violent cataclysm; although the contemporaries of Alaric and Romulus Augustulus were scarcely aware of what was happening, that a world was dropping into chaos — yet no civilization suffered more complete obliteration. It was the most appalling catastrophy in history. Human civilization seemingly powerful and securely established, embracing the known world in one organised, peaceful, prosperous society was completely blotted out. . . .

The depth of that ruin is not generally realized in its full horror. . . . From the fifth to the tenth century Europe lay sunk in a night of barbarism which grew darker and darker. It was a barbarism more awful and horrible than that of the primitive savage, for it was the decomposing body of what had been a great civilization. . . .[11]

Such contrasting opinions on the same period by intelligent writers serve to emphasize the inadvisability of a dogmatic attitude concerning the dark age. The best scholars of the historical profession are inclined to take a middle ground. The following balanced characterization is representative.

The middle ages was . . . not a long, level stretch of 1000 years with mankind stationary . . . but a downward and then an upward slope, on both of which the forces that make for civilization may be seen at work. . . . The fifth century politically introduces not so much the history of medieval as of *modern Europe.* . . . The barbarians destroyed much, but much survived. . . . The dark ages was a reality, but the traditional middle ages are a myth.[12]

Another recent historian adopts the broad viewpoint that;

11

the period from Augustine to Abelard was long known as the dark ages, but scholars have come to realize that the age was by no means devoid of great intellects or real cultural interests. . . . First rate intelligences worked hard over the crude materials at hand.[13]

One of the most interesting opinions comes from a learned contributor to our most up to date modern compendium, the new *Encyclopedia Britannica.* He writes as follows:

The centuries following the collapse of the Roman Empire are in an especial sense dark through the insufficiency of historical evidence.[14]

This passage it will be noted, tends to transfer the responsibility for the darkness of the early middle ages from the people of that day to the scholars of modern times, who are " in the dark " as to many of the achievements of that era. All in all, the trend of the most reliable opinion of our day seems to be toward the view that the early middle ages were not centuries of primitive violence or stagnation, but of cultural progress.

So far we have said nothing specifically concerning early medieval science or medicine. These subjects have a very important relationship to the problem of revaluing the early middle ages in the light of recent knowledge. The extent and quality of the darkness in the dark age have been reduced not merely by researches in the general culture of certain progressive centuries, but also by researches which show the continuity of various phases of civilization throughout the entire period. That is, the dark age has been studied not only by cross sections, but also longitudinally. For instance, students of late Roman literature, art, music, and economic life are led without perceptible break in continuity, deep into the middle ages. Likewise, he who seeks the roots of modern literature, art, music and economic life must perforce dip back into these early centuries. As an example we cite the findings in one field of medical history. It is a well-known fact that medical prescriptions of the same type exist in the writings of the centuries from Galen and Pliny the Elder, to Oribasius and Marcellus Empiricus, in late imperial times. That is, there was continuity in classical pharmacy up to the very threshold of the middle ages. But Dr. Sigerist and one of his students have published collections of similar prescriptions dating from the ninth, tenth, eleventh, and twelfth centuries, and from regions as far removed as Scotland, Switzerland and Italy.[15] Their conclusion is now generally accepted to the effect that there was in Western Europe throughout the middle ages a common body of medical remedies based on classical collections.

There are similar trends and viewpoints concerning other phases of early medieval development; all of which indicates that there is " pay dirt " in the early middle ages. Of this faith are many students of medical history.

On the other hand, a large percentage of medical historians and most students of medicine hold to the traditional opinion that the dark age was very dark. Like myself, many a casual reader must have been surprised to find a prominent American medical journal giving a large portion of one of its numbers to a ludicrous " Rhymed Outline of Medical History," written by a physician. Out of approximately fifty brief chapters, just one, containing eight lines, was devoted to the ten centuries of medieval medicine. In the following light-hearted manner the author dismissed the subject.

> Throughout the middle ages
> Medicine was devoid of sages
> Save for one leap from inferno—
> (Wisdom nurtured at Salerno

doctors on the early M.A

By helping hospital and nurse—)
Those years could otherwise be worse.
The Black Death, that most potent pest
Put sixty million souls to rest.[16]

Having thus put the middle ages to rest, the poet-physician continued with page after page of similarly childish history concerning modern medicine. But, after all, such trivialities are not so dangerous as the unintentional aberrations of the medical men who write serious history. No one who has read any considerable number of these works needs further proof of the fact that many writers are " in the dark " as to the dark age. It is not, however, our purpose to belabor physicians or medical historians for their failure to treat any particular epoch with the proper respect. We would instead set forth the medical generalizations that are current concerning the dark age with the hope of illustrating and explaining, first of all, the conflicts in opinion, and secondly the characteristically unsympathetic attitude that prevails toward the period in question. This will in turn serve as a background for the presentation of a few facts concerning medicine during this era.

With the example of the older school of historians before them, little wonder that most physicians and

untrained medical historians should have joined the
ranks of the pessimists and, after the fashion of
Gibbon considered the early middle ages as merely
" The Decline and Fall " of Graeco-Roman medical
science. As late as the year 1913, one of the world's
most famous physicians, lecturing on *The Evolution
of Modern Medicine*, gave the following characterization of the early middle ages.

There are waste places of the earth which fill one with
terror. . . . With this feeling we enter the Middle Ages.
Following the glory that was Greece and the grandeur that
was Rome, a desolation came upon the civilized world, in
which the light of learning burned low, flickering almost
to extinction. How came it possible that the gifts of
Athens and Alexandria were deliberately thrown away?
For three causes. The barbarians shattered the Roman
Empire to its foundations. When Alaric entered Rome in
410 A. D., ghastly was the impression made on the contemporaries; the Roman World shuddered in a titanic spasm
(Lindner). The land was a garden of Eden before them,
behind a howling wilderness, as is so graphically told in
Gibbon's great history. Many of the most important centers
of learning were destroyed, and for centuries Minerva and
Apollo forsook the haunts of men. . . .[17]

With only a trifle less of the melodramatic, the
lecturer went on to describe the devastating effects of

Christianity and the great plague of the sixth century. The most interesting factor in this lecturer's historical sketch is the fact that he took his ideas from the works of the historians of yesterday. This is neither the first nor the last instance in which historians have proved to be blind leaders of the blind into the pitfalls of the middle ages.

Others, writing more serious works of scholarship, have followed where Gibbon led. An eminent German of the epoch in which German scientific works won universal recognition, wrote a much quoted history of botany in which the following opinion was expressed.

During the time of Charles the Great and his closest successors there was practically no medicine . . . only here and there quacks who took the place of doctors. . . . The monks referred sick people to God's will, prayer, holy water, and the relics of the saints. . . . In the same deep sleep was medical study throughout the tenth and well into the second half of the eleventh century. . . . [18]

Others have expressed themselves in similarly pessimistic terms.

But this is not the whole story. There are medical historians who seem to believe in the adage " there is so much good in the worst." . . . The late Dr.

17

medical historians

Garrison, whose history of medicine has been for years the leading American handbook on the subject, was impressed with the " dreary stagnation " of the middle ages; its " bigotry, dogmatism, and mental inertia " and the " implicit belief in the miraculous healing power of saints and of holy relics." [19] But he was also aware of the new light that was being thrown on the subject. In a public address he once paid tribute to the work of scholars such as Sudhoff, Streeter, and Mrs. Dorothea Singer in illuminating the dark corners of the middle ages.[20] Even in the nineteenth century, the early middle ages had an occasional defender. In *An Epitome of the History of Medicine*, written just before the turn of the century, the following appeared.

Down to the seventh century in Rome there were court-archiaters . . . and in each large city popular archiaters formed a college charged with sanitary matters, the instruction and examination of candidates, and gratuitious services to the poor. . . . In the time of Charlemagne, for instance, the colleges of the cathedrals and even some of the monasteries taught medicine in a very limited way. Priest, abbots and bishops became court physicians. The monks of Monte Cassino . . . enjoyed for a long time a reputation for medical skill. . . .[21]

Earlier in the same century Dr. Charles Daremberg,

the most eminent French authority on medical history, lashed furiously at the historians of his own day.

Our modern historians [said he] . . . have summarized the history of the early middle ages with the two words, ignorance and superstition, but it is to them and not to the centuries which they have misunderstood that these words belong. . . . Until one has searched the manuscripts and found nothing he has no right to speak of ignorance. . . . There was no break in the medieval tradition. The barbarians were the immediate and direct heirs of Rome.[32]

Not many historians of our day accept this dictum in its entirety, but most of them are inclined to give the dark age a fair and sympathetic hearing. Dr. Castiglioni asserts that " critical studies have shown that . . . wisdom and civilization were not blotted out in Italy." [23] In similar fashion, Professor Lynn Thorndike writes that " apparently at no time during the period of the barbarian invasions and the early medieval centuries did medical practice or literature cease entirely in the West . . . physicians were fairly numerous and in good repute and medieval Christians at no time depended entirely upon the healing virtues of relics of saints or other miraculous powers." [24] Dr. James Walsh, in his all too brief survey of " Early Medieval Medicine," suggests that both the early and the later centuries of the middle ages "contain contributions to medicine that are worthy of consideration, and nearly always the writings that have been preserved for us demonstrate the fact that men were thinking for themselves as well as studying the Greek writers, and were making observations and garnering significant personal experience." [25]

So far as opinions are concerned, it seems that the most reliable of recent medical historians are quite definitely favorable in their attitude toward the early middle ages. It is sometimes asserted that this is merely another instance of the spirit of the twentieth century; an age that must dethrone the heroes of the past and enthrone its villains. But those who appreciate the dark age are not faddists; they are invariably the historians who, like Dr. Daremberg, have studied it most carefully. Is it possible that close contact lends enchantment to this barbaric epoch? One who knows and loves the middle ages has described his own experience in language which perhaps expresses the reaction of most individuals on coming into close contact with things medieval.

The early middle ages are often called the dark ages. I have been in Ravenna. I saw the golden light reflected

from the mosaics. I saw Jesus Christ, the good sheperd throned like Apollo, or like the *Roi Soleil* among his herds. I saw many romance cathedrals and found little darkness.[26]

With so many eminent scholars expressing themselves favorably concerning the dark age, it is surprising to find that the average student, professor, and doctor has a hopelessly antiquated concept of early medieval medicine. From actual tests, questionnaires, and informal conversations extending over a number of years I have come to the conclusion that most people cling very firmly to the handy titles and epoch designations which were drilled into them by patient school teachers during their impressionable adolescent years. This means that they are at least a quarter of a century behind the latest findings of scholarship, for it takes years for new information to seep down to the text book, high school, and gram mar-grade levels. Many an educated man's concel tion of the early middle ages is merely an amplifi image of the term dark age, the sole remnant youthful acquisitions in a history class.

Thus it is that the average medical student physician, with an education in history often sisting of a mere smattering of catch words, thought pattern of early medieval medicine th

21

marked variance with that of up to date medical historians. The average trained mind proceeds somewhat in this fashion; those were dark ages, therefore they must have been barbaric in their medical practice, and since they were barbaric how could they have had any intelligent physicians? Because of their simple Christian faith, most medieval folk resorted for healing to saint's relics and superstitious charms. Furthermore they were misled by medical quacks, old witches with their herbs and incantations, midwives, and blood-letting barbers. Such is the average mental image of medieval medicine. So prevalent is the tendency to deduce from the name of the period a distorted idea of conditions therein, that many historians would gladly dispense with traditional epoch designations such as dark age. Meanwhile intelligent students, and especially writers, might well follow the suggestion of a recent botanical historian who wrote that it is high time for scholars " to cease to perpetuate their own hereditary prejudices "; instead they should turn to " making intelligent use of the scattered fragments of historical information " that are now available.[27] And it is high time that we turn to the scattered fragments of information concerning dark age medical practice, and let them speak

for themselves concerning medicine in that little known period. We shall limit our attention to that portion of the middle ages extending from the sixth to the eleventh century. This somewhat drab, but rather important age was that in which Western civilization took shape. It began with the Germanic occupation of the disintegrated empire of the West, and ended just before the First Crusade.

We turn now to a few citations from the literature of various regions and centuries of this age. These will serve to illustrate the fact that there were two distinct types of medicine; supernatural and human. Supernatural healing included first the reliance upon Christian saints and their relics, secondly Christian-pagan charms and magical incantations. Human medicine consisted chiefly of empirical methods of healing, notably by means of drugs, surgery, and diet.

Supernatural healing by means of relics and the like is by far the most prominent aspect of medicine miracle as presented in the chronicles and religious biographies of the early middle ages. But in this literature such factors were given an exaggerated importance. The authors were churchmen whose major purpose was the pious edification of their people. Therefore

23

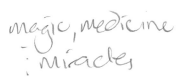

magic, medicine
miracles

they emphasized religious healing. For the earlier centuries the most noteworthy examples are Bishop Gregory of Tours (died 593) and Pope Gregory the Great (died 604).

Bishop Gregory of Tours outdid all medieval writers in both quantity and quality of miracle tales. His accounts are so vivid that they have tended to dominate the picture of early medieval medicine as portrayed by modern writers. Inasmuch as we shall make detailed use of Gregory's works later in treating of the Merovingian age, at this point we shall cite only one case, that of a woman who was afflicted by demons so that her tongue was paralysed. Gregory related that:

The people tried an appliance of herbs and verbal incantations, but were not able by medical skill to allay the malady . . . our daughter [Gregory's niece, Eustachia] coming to the sick woman and seeing her with the stupid herb dressing, poured oil from the holy sepulchre into her mouth. As a result the sick woman began to convalesce.[28]

This quotation illustrates three outstanding attitudes found in the writings of Gregory, and many another medieval churchman. In the first place, disease was attributed to sin or demons; secondly, human medi-

24

cine was considered of no avail; and finally saintly intervention usually effected a cure.

Pope Gregory, although he wrote less than Bishop Gregory concerning medicine, had no less faith in miracles. In his *Dialogues*, a collection of stories concerning the lives and miracles of the Italian Saints, he related many pious tales of men who were delivered from demons or raised from the dead. He like Bishop Gregory was a firm believer in miraculous cures.[29]

In most of the Saints' lives written during the middle ages, healing was treated after this same fashion, as a supernatural intervention. But in the chronicles and other less pious sources there eventually developed a more natural interpretation. The change is apparent in the works of the Venerable Bede who lived and wrote in an English monastery over a century after the two Gregories. In Bede's *History of the Church of England* there are numerous tales of miraculous healing. The accounts of ailments cured by means of potions made from chips of St. Oswald's cross, or dust from the ground where he had died,[30] are strikingly similar to Bishop Gregory's accounts of the wonder working powers of St. Martin's relics at Tours. But there is this difference; as stated by an English authority on Bede: " It is noticeable that of the many marvels which Bede records, he does not give one on his own knowledge, and his lives of the first five abbots of his own monastery contain no notice of a single miracle." [31] If this interpretation be justified, and it is certainly in keeping with the general character of Bede's scholarship, it exemplifies a rather marked change of attitude among early medieval intellectuals.

The records from the Carolingian Age are even less insistent on the miraculous in healing. To be sure, saintly biographies such as that of St. Gall, contain accounts of " demons cast out, sick persons restored to health, deaf ears opened, eyes freed from darkness, and the silence of the dumb broken, and the impotence of the palsied relieved," [32] all by divine intervention. But the earlier intolerance of human medicine is conspicuously absent, even from the writings of the clergy. For instance, there is Rabanus Maurus, Abbot of Fulda and Archbishop of Mainz. He was quite as conservative a churchman as either of the Gregories, but in his *de Universo*, a handbook written for the use of clerical students, he devoted an entire section to medicine, describing the various aspects of non-religious healing without any animus. His only pious aberration was a belief in sin as a cause for disease. Writing concerning soreness of the eyes he concluded that " he is blear-eyed who is dragged down by earthly lust and does not lift the eyes of his mind in Heavenly contemplation." [33] Later we shall hear more concerning Rabanus' tendency to moralize concerning medicine. From the Alpine regions during the same century comes a most vivid and amusing account which illustrates the manner in which Carolingian clergymen emphasized the physical aspects of illness, not however without adding a moral precept concerning divine retribution. Abbot Walafrid Strabo of Reichenau, in describing the manner in which God punished a bishop of Constance for his evil life, told of his final illness as follows:

He entered the church of St. Gall as if to pray and stationed himself before the altar of the Saint, and there . . . this man received condign recompense . . . for the sufferings he had sworn to inflict on others. For suddenly his bowels began to seethe like a saucepan over a fire and he was seized by such terrible gripings that he could never have left the church without aid; and (I am ashamed to tell it) he yielded to the promptings of nature in a way that was highly offensive to the nostrils of all present. He was thrust out of the church without delay and at his own desire was placed in a vehicle and left the monastery. And so he took his departure, seated on a chamber pot and undergoing the most unnatural purgations. He was taken to the monastery of Reichenau of which he was abbot at the time; there his malady became worse and the stench of his person became so intolerable that hardly any of his attendants could render their wanted services. Thus punished for his deeds a few days later he breathed forth his spirit from the foul sewer of his body. . . . [34]

Throughout the ensuing centuries the shift of emphasis from the miraculous to the human aspects of illness and healing continued. To be sure, churchmen and pious folk never completely divested themselves of the idea that disease was a divine visitation. But the contrast between the concepts of the age of the Gregories and those of the later centuries is sharp and convincing. This will be more evident as we consider the various phases of human medicine.

The second phase of supernatural healing was a combination of pagan and Christian superstition. In Roman folk-medicine, incantations, charms, and magic played an important part. The pages of Pliny's *Natural History*, and Marcellus Empiricus' handbook of medicine bear ample evidence of the fact. Professor Thorndike, an authority on the history of magic, even contends that Pliny's work

magic

28

contained a higher proportion of magic than the sixth century *Etymologies* of the Christian bishop, Isidore of Seville.[35] The fact seems to be that the Christian abhorrence of things pagan tended to eliminate from early medieval medicine much of Roman superstition. Isidore himself condemned pagan practices such as ligatures, suspensions, and incantation, on the ground that they were the work of the Devil and were contrary to the art of medicine.[36] Nevertheless medieval folk-healers continued to use magical lore, under cover of Christian prayers and often with the sign of the cross. In similar fashion Germanic and Celtic superstitions persisted in the Christian world of medicine. Germanic practice was highly charged with sorcery, based for the most part on the principle of driving out the demons which caused the ailment. This was often done by touching the patient with the blood of a sacrificed animal, or by runes marked on bits of wood, or by magical stones and amulets. Magic also invaded the field of pharmacy, through the medium of certain rituals which accompanied the collecting of herbs or the concocting of drugs.

In general, however, there was surprisingly little of superstitious practice in early medieval medicine.

The narrative sources contain an occasional reference to *harioli* and other types of medicine men. Extant medical manuscripts from this age contain medical treatises and collections of medieval prescriptions in both of which there is an occasional magical formula or prayer. For eye trouble, for instance, the following incantation was used; " I adjure you spots, that you go away and recede from, and be destroyed from the eye of the servant of God." [37] For the bite of an adder one might be advised to drink holy water in which a black snail had been washed. But such remedies make up a comparatively small portion of the subject matter of the manuscripts. Only in England where, in the opinion of Doctor Singer, the existence of a vernacular language made possible early written records of the medical practices of the common folk, do we find any great quantity of actual superstition. Excellent examples of this literature are available in Reverend Oswald Cockayne's *Leechdoms, Wortcunnings and Starcraft of Early England.*[38]

Furthermore the accounts of divine healing and superstition do not tell the entire story of early medieval medicine. Although the hand of God (and other supernatural agencies) was the major theme of most writers of the period when they concerned themselves with medical affairs, they also presented many evidences concerning the hand of the physician; that is, concerning practical or empirical medicine. This ranged from the simplest midwifery to the surgery and urine analysis of royal physicians. Although much of this practice was close to the level of ignorant superstition, some of it was surprisingly intelligent and progressive. We shall consider the empirical phases of medicine under the three categories commonly employed in medieval treatises; namely pharmacy, diet, and surgery.

Of the three, pharmacy was by far the most prominent. It comprised the collecting of herbs and other simple substances, and the compounding of complex remedies. Everywhere, in the contemporary sources, simple drugs and compound cure-alls, comparable to the patent medicines of our day, are much in evidence. In the hand books of remedies, called *antidotaria* or *receptaria*, are lists of medical prescriptions which present a strange mingling of superstition and intelligence, of folk medicine and classical pharmacy. Much of this material belonged to the great body of empirical remedies which took shape during late Roman times in the works attributed to Pliny Secundus, Theodore Priscian, Cassius Felix,

Apuleius, Sextus Placitus, and Marcellus Empiricus.
This included not only antidotes, electuaries, laxatives, theriacs and various kinds of potions, but also
ointments, plasters, powders, pills, and other such
compounds.

The very titles of many of the remedies indicate
the unscientific nature of the medical practice of the
day. There were prescriptions recommended to make
a woman conceive, to prevent conception, to improve
the memory, to prevent drunkenness, to eliminate
frightful dreams, for falling hair, for pimples,
" against a woman's chatter," and even " for foul
stench under the armpits." [39] The materials used in
concocting remedies also reveal much of superstition.
In addition to herbs of various kinds, urine, the ex-
cretion of animals, powdered earth-worms, and portions of the organs of animals might be used. For
example, the testicles of roosters were used as a
remedy for impotency.[40]

Weird though the dark age remedies were, it must
be noted that they were by no means a peculiarly
medieval invention. Many of the most offensive
prescriptions can be traced back through late imperial times to the early Romans, the Greeks, and
even the Egyptians. Who is there who would not,

at first glance, attribute the following to some ignorant medieval practitioner; " If you save the urine of a person who eats cabbage habitually and bathe the patient in it he will be quickly healed." The same writer recommended cabbage mixed with ham scrapings, beets, fern, mussels, scorpions, snails and lentils as an excellent purgative. As a matter of fact, these and many other curious prescriptions appear in a treatise *Concerning Agriculture* written in the heyday of the Roman Republic by one of the most intelligent of farmer-statesmen, Marcus Porcius Cato.[41] It seems probable that much of the same sort of medical remedies has been prevalent in every age from ancient Egypt to the frontier days of American history. The following incident is an interesting and vivid illustration of this fact.

Once upon a time a king, while shaving, fell unconscious in his bedroom. The following treatment was employed by the royal physicians. A pint of blood was extracted from his right arm; then eight ounces from the left shoulder; next an emetic, two physics, and an enema consisting of 15 substances. Then his head was shaved and a blister raised on the scalp. To purge the brain a sneezing powder was given; then cowslip powder to strengthen it. Meanwhile more emetics, soothing drinks, and more bleeding; also a plaster of pitch and pigeon dung applied to the royal feet. Not to leave anything undone, the following substances were taken internally: melon seeds, manna, slippery elm, black cherry water, extract of lily of the valley, peony, lavender, pearls dissolved in vinegar, gentian root, nutmeg, and finally 40 drops of extract of human skull. As a last resort bezoar stone was employed. But the royal patient died.[42] A perfect example, one might say, of the murderous effects of medieval medical superstition. But this occurred in modern times, a little over two centuries ago. The unfortunate patient was Charles II, King of England. The middle ages, however, and particularly the earlier centuries had a higher proportion of the primitive, and much less of so-called " scientific " pharmacy than the preceding and succeeding ages.

Before leaving the subject of pharmacy we may take note of the fact that the majority of the early medieval prescriptions, though primitive, were reasonably intelligent. Usually they were remedies for ordinary ailments such as fevers, headaches, intestinal difficulties, toothache, sore eyes, wounds, and bites of snakes or mad dogs. The ingredients most used were herbs.

The animal substances, bodily excretions, and other revolting materials, which impress the modern reader so vividly, were not used in the majority of prescriptions. The following are examples of the simple remedies which one finds constantly in manuscripts. " For headache take the root of peony mixed with oil of roses. When thoroughly mixed soak a piece of linen in it and apply constantly to the place where the pain is. Without doubt it will help." [43] And again, " For toothache mix vinegar with oil and sulphur and put in the mouth of the sufferer." [44] Such remedies had little effect, but it has been estimated that they were much less harmful than the mercurial and other metallic remedies which were used in the early modern centuries.

science can hurt

There are those who with laudable stubborness refuse to accept such citations from manuscripts as actual evidence of the medical practice of the early middle ages. With reason they assert that such prescriptions may have been mere transcriptions of classical works, copied as a part of the mechanical task of a monastic scribe, never to be used by a medieval doctor. But the manner in which the prescriptions were scribbled in margins or blank spaces suggests that they were acquired and recorded deliberately, for some special purpose. Further evidence of the fact that such prescriptions were actually used is found in the fact that contemporary writers compiled their own collections. In addition to the many anonymous antidotaries and receptaries,[45] there were two ninth century compendia composed by Abbot Bertharius of Monte Cassino, and the antidotary of Donnolo, an Italian Jew of the tenth century. Most interesting of all, however, is the *Hortulus* of Abbot Walafrid Strabo of Reichenau. This learned Carolingian churchman combined materials from classical herbals with information gained in his own day by practical experience, recording it all in a simple poetical form that could be easily remembered. His was clearly a book for everyday use. And the remedies therein contained were for the most part as sane and sensible as most of the folk-prescriptions of ancient and early modern times. A few examples taken at random will illustrate this point. For dyspepsia a concoction of poppy was recommended, in the following sprightly couplet:

> The belching of wind it will quickly allay,
> And take the foul taste in your mouth right away.[46]

Parsley was suggested as a remedy for biliousness, even though the sufferer were a king.

Suppose now His Majesty bilious feels,
Mix vinegar, parsley, and water in one;
Then the belly recovers and griping is done.[47]

Walafrid had sure, though simple cures for all sorts of ailments, including bladder trouble, colds, and festered wounds. He believed firmly in the virtues of radish.

A piece of this hot-flavored root bitten off
And chewed, will expell the most shattering cough.[48]

For vocalists he prescribed peppermint, insisting that

According to singers one kind will dispell
All harshness and make the voice clear as a bell.
For continuing rasping which dries up the throat;
Drink some peppermint—it will enliven your note.[49]

For head wounds he advised as follows:

Clap a poultice of betony leaves on the spot
Then watch how the strength of the herb is revealed
As the sore disappears and the wound is soon healed.[50]

The essentially practical character of Walafrid's book is illustrated by a prescription which could serve two purposes. If bitten by a poisonous snake one should

Take a pestle and beat up a lily quite fine,
And drink the juice mixed with Falernian wine.

> The rest of the leaves that are bruised, you may place
> On a pimple or spot that disfigures your face.[51]

We quote one final prescription which may illustrate either the empirical or the superstitious aspects of early pharmaceutical practice; but one thing is certain, it reveals a sense of humor that is rare. In praising the virtues of horehound Walafrid said:

> Again if your stepmother bears you ill will
> And mixes a poisonous aconite pill
> In your food, and rejoices to see you look sad,
> As you swallow the drug and begin to feel bad
> Never worry, but drink of a cup of this herb,
> Your stepmother's evil designs it will curb.[52]

For doubting souls who might demand proof that medieval practitioners actually used pharmaceutical materials, it may be said also that the narrative sources contain references to potions, pills, ointments, and salves used for healing. A famous history of the monastery of St. Gall mentions " a most learned monk " named Iso who had cured lepers, paralytics, and even blind folk with " the ointments which he made." [53] In the letters of Fulbert of Chartres we shall have occasion to note in detail further examples of this sort of practice.[54]

Surgery, the second of the three major divisions

of human medicine, at first glance has little to recommend it. Most prominent was the process of cupping or blood-letting. It was employed constantly for all sorts of ailments, especially fevers. Sometimes the results were admittedly precarious; early medieval literature contains references to the dangerous swellings that followed the operation. Many a person in medieval times must have been bled to death. Blood-letting, like healing by means of drugs, was considerably influenced by superstition. There was a widely prevalent idea to the effect that it was dangerous, if not fatal to bleed people at certain unlucky seasons. This precaution, like so many other medieval practices, was an inheritance from classical or even earlier times. The name, " Egyptian Days " applied to this kind of medical taboo, suggests its origin. But during the early middle ages the superstitious aspects were magnified. Elaborate calendars were drawn up indicating the unlucky days not only for blood-letting but also for cathartics, and for taking certain types of food and drink.[55] In other respects blood-letting was conducted according to more sane principles. There were in most early medieval compendia brief treatises which contained explicit instructions concerning the places and methods for tapping the veins.[56]   Occasionally a warning was given against excessive bleeding.

Nowhere in the literature of the early middle ages is there any hint that blood-letting was performed by any other than the regular physicians. This ·is of importance in the face of the almost universal opinion of our day that throughout the middle ages blood-letting was performed by barbers. According to Alcuin and Walafrid Strabo this type of medical practice was carried on by the *medici*.[57] The projected monastic infirmary at St. Gall, which had special rooms for bleeding, was manned by regular physicians, with no mention of any other type of practitioner.[58] At Chartres and other North French centers, it was not until late in the eleventh century that *rasators* and *sanguinators* began to appear.[59] Late medieval physicians seem to have felt that blood-letting and pharmacy were beneath their professional dignity; but during the earlier centuries the *medici* were general practitioners, without benefit of barber-surgeon or apothecary.

Surgery of a higher order than blood-letting, though seldom given any prominence in the sources, existed. From sixth-century France there are several instances which will be considered later. At about the same time, in Spain a bishop of Merida was said to have performed a Caesarian operation.[60] From St. Gall in the ninth century we have a similar case. Fourteen days ahead of nature's schedule, according to the chronicler's account, " an infant was cut out of the mother's body and wrapped in the fat of a newly killed pig." [61] It is, of course, obvious that there was during this warlike age considerable military surgery, such as the amputation of limbs. For instance, in the list of fines for deeds of violence in the law codes of the seventh and eighth centuries there are brief, but illuminating references to surgical treatments and instruments for head-wounds.[62] One of the tenth century chronicles also makes reference to an operation on a Saxon monk who was suffering from severe pains in the head,[63] and Walafrid Strabo's *Hortulus* contains remedies for the healing of head wounds and the prevention of scars.[64] There is, however, no evidence of anything but the simplest methods. The surgical instruments mentioned in the sources and the discoveries by archaeologists reveal only primitive instruments and linen bandages.[65]

Somewhat closely related to surgery was the practice of cauterization. It was employed in the sixth century for the elimination of diseased tissues in both humans and animals.[66] From this period until the eleventh century there is very little mention of cauterization. Meanwhile quite a different usage developed. This was the application of the cautery iron at certain places for the relief of certain general ailments. The manuscripts of the later centuries contain elaborate treatises on the subject, with illustrations of human bodies marked with red spots to indicate the places at which the iron was to be applied.[67] Often the member cauterized had no apparent relationship to the ailment. The cauterization of wounds was more intelligently handled.

Diet or regimen as it was often called, was apparently the least important of the three types of non-religious healing. There was, however, some effort to control or prevent disease by means of food, drink, and other normal regulations of the body. We know that through the medium of sixth century Ostrogothic Italy, classical ideas concerning diet were made available to the Germanic people of the West. In one instance it came about thus: Anthimus, a Greek who had been exiled from Constantinople, came to Italy where he served as royal physician to Theodoric the Ostrogoth. He was sent as an ambassador to the court of the Frankish King, Theodoric, for whom he wrote a treatise on diet which bears the following ponderous title; *A Letter of Anthimus, the Illustrious Man, Count and Legate, to the Most Glorious King, Theodoric of the Franks, Concerning the Observance of Foods.*[68] Here, as Valentine Rose expressed it, a dietary regula " was written by a *Greek* physician, in *Latin*, for a *Germanic* King." [69] In his introduction Anthimus suggested that

in the first place man's health depends on proper foods; for if he eats well prepared foods his digestion is good. But if they are not well cooked, trouble develops in the stomach and abdomen, generating bad humors, ulcers, and severe belching. Whereupon fumes ascend to the head, and scotomatica and eye troubles result. . . .

He who observes the proper diet will not have to resort to other medicaments.

And the same is true of drinks. . . .

Above all, moderation is necessary.[70]

The author then proceeds to 94 paragraphs of advice concerning the various kinds of meats, eggs, fish, fowl, milk, cheese, butter, vegetables, and fruits. He suggested certain foods as correctives for certain ailments and urged in particular that one eat only carefully prepared food. Bread, for instance, should be light, not sour, and well baked.

Anthimus' treatise was based on classical works; in fact it bears a strong resemblance to certain portions of book II of Hippocrates, περὶ διαίτης.[71] But it was eminently practical in form and language, and was actually written down to the level of Germanic Latin. This fact, in part, answers the inevitable question; what indication is there that such materials were ever used during the early middle ages? There is also corroboratory evidence in the copies and epitomes of this treatise, extant in ninth and tenth century manuscripts. For example, in a tenth century manuscript we find a very brief epitome entitled " What Theodoric King of the Franks *used* and observed." [72] If Anthimus' treatise was being copied and epitomized three centuries after it was written, it would seem that it must have been " used and observed " during that time. A hint of this very thing comes from the *Life of Charles the Great*, in which Einhard reported that the emperor was very particular about his diet; was very moderate in drinking, and when sick abstained from food.[73] Cassiodorus, minister of state of Theodoric the Ostrogoth, whom Anthimus served as royal physician, left to posterity a form letter that had been used for the instruction of the chief *archiater*. Therein, the physician was urged, among other things to control the king's diet; "weary us if you wish *with fasting*, and make us do the opposite of what we desire; all of this is your prerogative," ordered the king.[74] It seems evident that Germanic kings were interested in dietary regulations and that considerably more attention was given to the subject during the early centuries than is apparent from the general narrative sources.[75]

Although pharmacy, surgery, and diet were the three recognized fields of early medieval medicine, there were other types of medical practice that are worthy of mention. It seems that an occasional physician was expert in diagnosis and urine analysis. That such ability was rare is evident from the reputation which it brought. A case in point is that of a famous monastic physician of St. Gall during the tenth century. Notker Balbus, also called *medicus* and *doctor*, was reputed to have been "a man of great knowledge," and one who "frequently performed wonders of healing that were unbelievable." One of the favorite accounts of his wonder-working ability concerned urine analysis. It seems that he was about to examine the Duke of Bavaria. As a trick, to test Notker, the Duke substituted for his own urine that of a woman who was pregnant. But

Notker after making his examination, without any apparent sign of suspicion made the solemn announcement that " God is about to bring to pass an unheard of event; within thirty days the Duke will give birth to a child." Whereupon the Duke was said to have blushed; but he insisted that the triumphant physician continue in his service.[76] It might also be noted that the early middle ages had manuscript treatises concerning urine analysis.[77]

Notker's accuracy in diagnosis was also lauded in another story concerning a man who was troubled with a nasal hemorrhage. From the smell of the blood, Notker predicted that within three days he would break out with smallpox, but refused to prevent it, asserting that he could do so but it would cause death. As he predicted the patient had smallpox but was so effectively treated that there was not a single pock mark left on his face.[78] Almost as interesting as the medical cures of Notker is the pride which the monastic chroniclers took in his exploits. This is far cry from Gregory of Tours' unending hymn of hate against human medicine.[79]

And now we turn from the practice to the practitioners of the medical art. In our survey of the various types of medicine in the early middle ages, we have found the clergy, and particularly the monks, occupying the most prominent place. This brings up the question as to the relative accuracy of the idea that this was a period of distinctly *clerical* medicine. An intelligent answer to this problem necessitates some comprehension of the extent of medical practice among the laity. In spite of the scant publicity given to lay physicians in the contemporary clerical-controlled sources, we have, especially for Italy, considerable fragmentary evidence of their activity. Under the Ostrogothic regime of the early sixth century there was a well regulated system of public doctors, including a group of superior physicians called *archiatri*, and a royally appointed " Count of *Archiatri*." The form letter for the appointment and instruction of this official, reads in part as follows:

The physician helps us when all other helpers fail. By his art he finds out things about a man of which he himself is ignorant; and his prognosis of a case, though founded on reason, seems to the ignorant like a prophecy. . . .

They [the physicians] ought not to quarrel. At the beginning of their exercise of the art they take a sort of priestly oath to hate wickedness and to love purity. Take then this rank of *Comes Archiatrorum*, and have the dis-

tinguished honour of presiding over so many skilled practitioners and of moderating their disputes. . . .

Leave it to the clumsy men to ask their patients if they
have had a good sleep; if the pain has left them. Do you
rather incline the patient to ask you about his own malady,
showing him that you know more about it than he does.
The patient's pulse, the patient's urine, tell a skilled physician the whole story of his disease. . . . [80]

In spite of the insinuation as to the quarrelsome-
ness of certain of the physicians, it is evident from
this letter that Ostrogothic Italy was favorable to the
lay profession. Alexander of Tralles, the greatest
Greek physician of the sixth century, is thought to
have lived, practiced, and perhaps taught medicine
in Rome for a time either during or just after the
period of the Ostrogothic rule.[81] Later in the century, even under the barbaric Lombards there was
some legal provision for the fees of physicians who
cared for wounded persons.[82]

In Transalpine lands also, there are occasional
evidences of the persistence of the Roman type of
municipal physician, and of the recognition by the
Germanic conquerors of a professional medical class
that was non-clerical. For the Frankish realm we
shall consider later the detailed references to *archiatri*
and other lay physicians.[83] It seems clear that the

profession did not enjoy as favorable a status as in Italy. Whereas Theodoric the Ostrogoth is known to have intervened to revise an unjust legal decision against an Italian physician,[84] in Frankland even the *archiatri* were sometimes plundered with impunity, or executed for their failure to cure a royal patient.

With the exception of Italy, throughout the West after the sixth and seventh centuries the medical activities of the laity appear to have been overshadowed by those of the clergy. In Italy these centuries mark the shadowy period of the beginning of Salernitan medicine. Without raising the question of the relative importance of classical-Roman or Christian-Benedictine influences in the history of Salerno, we may with safety cite this center as an example of the continuity of the lay medical profession in Italy. There is also some evidence of lay physicians in certain municipal records of this period.[85] There is a strong tendency today to accept the theory of the continuity of lay institutions, such for instance as municipal schools, throughout medieval Italy. It is our opinion that the lay profession of medicine also had an unbroken existence throughout this period of Italian history.

On the other hand, everywhere, as time passed

the clergy became more and more active in medicine.

It is the Italian monasteries that furnish the outstanding examples. Here, during the first half of the sixth century, Benedict of Nursia worked out the monastic system in which we find the first faint beginnings of monastic medicine. The Benedictine rule provided for the establishment of an infirmary in each monastery, and asserted that "the care of the sick is to be placed above and before every other duty ... the infirmarian must be thoroughly reliable, known for his piety and diligence, solicitous for his charges." [86] It must be noted, however, that this service was simple and that it was primarily for the fellow monks, not for the populace at large. The early Benedictines were ascetics, not medical missionaries.

Far more important than Benedict in the making of monastic medicine, was Cassiodorus, a man who had spent most of his life in secular affairs. Shortly after the death of Benedict, Cassiodorus laid the foundation of what might have been a real medical science. In a book of instructions for the monks of his private monastery he stressed, after the manner of Benedict, the importance of " caring for the bodies of the brethren who have entered the sacred places."

But, unlike Benedict he provided medical books from which they might learn the classical art of healing.

Learn therefore (he urged) the nature of herbs and study diligently the ways to combine the various species for human health; but do not place your entire hope on herbs nor seek to restore health only by human counsels. Since medicine was created by God, and since it is he who gives help and restores life, turn to him. And if the language of the Greeks is unknown to you, you have the herb book of Dioscorides which describes with surprising exactness the herbs of the field. After that read Hippocrates and Galen in Latin translations; that is to say the *Therapeutics* of the latter which he addressed to the philosopher Glauco; and the work of an anonymous author, which as an examination shows is compiled from various authors; then the *Medicine* of Aurelius Caelius, the book of Hippocrates *On Herbs and Cures* and various other writings on the healing art which by God's help I have been able to procure for you in my library.[87]

This passage, the latter part of which is often quoted, indicates not only the intellectual interests of Cassiodorus, but also his reliance on the supernatural. He seems to have been, like Benedict, chiefly interested in the health of " the brethren." None the less, he set an intellectual ideal that had much influence on later monastic medicine. Unfortunately it was not emulated to any considerable degree by the Benedictines of his own day.

The medical achievements of the medieval clergy were destined to be a combination of the Benedictine ideal of brotherly service with Cassiodorus' plan for an intelligent comprehension of medicine based on the study of classical texts. But for several centuries the clergy took little active interest in human medicine. It was Ravenna and other non-monastic centers that took the lead in the translation of Greek medical texts and their transmission to the Latin West. It is believed that during the eighth century public readings of Hippocrates and Galen were held in Ravenna.[88] Furthermore, in the far away British Isles, during this era, medical information, both classical and native, was being compiled in the Anglo-Saxon language of the lay public.[89].

The first outstanding evidence of intelligent medical research in Benedict's own monastery of Monte Cassino comes from the ninth century when Abbot Bertharius compiled two medical works. Interestingly enough the monastic library has today a ninth century medical manuscript which is thought to be one of these compilations. It is a six hundred page manuscript containing lists of antidotes, of substitutions for drugs, of ailments and of remedies arranged according to diseases; also tables of weights and measures and synonyms for herbs. Then there are more serious treatises concerning fevers, urine, and the diagnosis of diseases; and as always a list of the months and days in which certain food and treatments should be avoided. Classical names such as Hippocrates and Galen are attached to some of the treatises. This manuscript is an excellent example of the type of compilation that was available in many early medieval libraries.[90]

Such was the case at the monastery of St. Gall on the Lake of Constance. Like Monte Cassino, St. Gall had medically minded abbots. In the ninth century Abbot Grimaldus was reported to have given a medical manuscript to the monastic library, and it was to him that Walafrid Strabo, abbot of nearby Reichenau, dedicated his *Hortulus*.[91] There are extant copies not only of medical manuscripts at St. Gall but also of early catalogues which list the medical books in the library at that time. For instance, in the ninth century catalogue one finds entries such as the following; " Three medical books, two large and one small; three medical books in quaternions." [92] In one of the early catalogues there are six medical works listed in a total of several hundred entries.[93] Today out of some 1700 medieval manuscripts about a dozen are from the early middle ages.[94] One or two of these can be dated as pre-Carolingian;[95] two of them were written in the insular Irish or Anglo-Saxon hand.[96] Most of the early medical manuscripts of St. Gall are, like that of Monte Cassino already described, compilations from classical treatises, collections of remedies, etc. In several of these manuscripts the subject matter is consolidated into large blocks of material, organized into books and chapters, with tables of contents for handy reference.[97]

But St. Gall had something more than manuscripts and theoretical knowledge. Here the monks seem to have combined the knowledge of classical medical literature with efficient medical equipment. We have the original ninth-century plan of an infirmary with efficiently arranged and adequate accomodations for several physicians and for ailing monks.[98] The infirmary was segregated from the rest of the monastic community. It was provided with a separate chapel, an open courtyard, heated and unheated rooms, a dormitory, dining room, kitchen, baths and numerous toilets. There were special wards for serious cases, rooms for blood-letting and purging, a pharmaceutical dispensary and separate rooms for the head physician, the other physicians, and the superintendent. At one corner of the infirmary enclosure was an herb garden with separate beds for sixteen varieties of plants.[99] If it was ever completed this infirmary had its own administrative staff, and a well planned set of buildings which provided for efficient medical service. On the other hand, there are indications that the treatment was very simple; merely herbal pharmacy, purging and bleeding. There was no apparent provision for complicated surgery. Nor was this a public hospital for outsiders; it was strictly monastic. The objection may be raised that the mere plan of a medical center does not prove its actual existence. But oddly enough, there are written records of well organized hospitals from sixth century Visigothic Spain and eleventh century Italy.[100] Furthermore, the medical practices indicated in the St. Gall plan are almost identical with the procedure outlined in a contemporary description of a Carolingian medical center; namely, a number of physicians, blood-letting, pharmacy, and (that which was peculiarly characteristic of the middle age), prayer for divine assistance.[101] By adding to these something of dietary regulations, cautery, surgical operations, and urine analysis, one has the sum total of the early medieval practice of medicine.

If we accept the contemporary sources as representative of the medical practice of this period, it is obvious that at the beginning of the early middle ages, while Roman influences were still strong, the laity were more active than the clergy. Later this situation was reversed, and after the seventh century, the monks were foremost, with the secular clergy and the laity very much in the background. The most noteworthy development in medicine was the changing attitude of the clergy. During the early centuries they endeavored to suppress human medicine as a dangerous rival of supernatural healing. But by virtue of the Christian principle of caring for the sick, and the medical knowledge gained from classical texts and practical experience, little by little the clergy came to appreciate human medicine. By the ninth and tenth centuries the monks were beginning to approve and publicize the medical achievements of members of their fraternity. Their superior control over the channels of literary communication enhanced considerably their well deserved medical fame. But already the secular clergy were attaining prominence in the medical realm, and by the end of the era we find them rivaling the monks.

If medical history is really a part of the history of civilization, it is concerned with mankind, not only at his moments of supreme achievements, but also in periods of retrogression. Medical historians may therefore with profit give careful consideration to periods such as the early middle ages. Here they may learn little concerning medical science, but much concerning mankind in a period of decline, recovery and growth. Here is to be found not only a portion of the ancient world in process of disintegration, but also a primitive Germanic people emerging from barbarism, and a Christian priesthood progressing from superstitious intolerance to scientific intelligence. Dr. Singer, the eminent English scholar, has defended medieval medical history on the ground that it is a study in the pathology of civilization.[102] But it is more than this; it is the birth and growth of a new civilization. Early medieval civilization consisted of two healthy elements, and one that was old and pathological. In the West, although classical civilization was sick unto death, much of it was preserved through its union with a vigorous young religion (Christianity) and a sturdy new race of rulers (the Germans). These two furnished the active elements by which a practically new civilization was created. The early middle age is a period in which the clergy, originally dedicated to supernatural healing, and the Germanic people, addicted to primitive folk medicine, slowly progressed to the point where they could appreciate classical medical science and apply more intelligently the results of their own practical experience. Western medicine, which in the sixth century was well toward the bottom of the ladder, by 1100 had made noteworthy progress. Far from being stagnant and unproductive, the " dark age " was an era of vigorous activity. Some of the definite stages of this progress can be seen in considerable detail in the medical history of France during this period.

II

MEDICINE IN MEROVINGIAN AND
CAROLINGIAN FRANCE

IN the first lecture of this series we followed a
two-fold purpose; an analysis of the changing
modern concept of the dark ages, and a survey of
certain general aspects of the medical practice prevailing in Western Europe during this era. We shall
now direct our attention to France; especially to the
northern regions, and finally to one of the most
notable medical centers, the cathedral school of
Chartres. Our general plan, it will be noted, is to
concentrate on successively smaller regions of the
West, ending with an intensive study of a restricted
center, which was preeminent in medical activities.

The land with which we are concerned was the
Gaul of Roman times. It comprised approximately
the region now known as France (which name we
shall employ). During the early middle ages this
expanse of territory was controlled by the Franks.
It was not one of the most progressive of the Germanic realms of the West; neither was it as destitute
of civilized life as England or the Germanies. In
short, France presents a more nearly average picture

of early medieval medicine than would Salernitan Italy or Saxon Germany.

A. THE MEROVINGIAN AGE

Our knowledge of French medicine during the Pre-Carolingian, or Merovingian age is particularly meager. There are very few historical chronicles and almost no other sources of information such as medical manuscripts. Truly this period, which comprises the sixth, seventh, and eighth centuries, might be spoken of as peculiarly dark because of the scarcity of our information concerning it. The few extant records are almost entirely religious in character; lives of the saints, ecclesiastical histories, and the like.[103] As might be expected, such sources contain very little medical information, and what there is has an unavoidable religious bias. One would hardly look for much evidence concerning early American medicine in a History of the United States by Brigham Young, or in the Life of Roger Williams by a Baptist clergyman; but it is exactly this sort of material on which we are forced to rely for our knowledge of French medicine during the Merovingian age. Most numerous are the pious biographies of holy men such as St. Martin of Tours. These were written by monks or priests and solely for the purposes of religious edification. The only detailed chronological account is the *History of the Franks* written by Gregory, Bishop of Tours.[104] There is little else save fragments of laws and minor treatises.

Due no doubt to the scantiness of evidence, most writers on medical history have been content to quote Gregory's most vivid tales of miracle healing and let the Merovingian age go at that. Unfortunately these are often interpreted as typical not only of his viewpoint but also of the general state of medicine in the early middle ages. The first assumption is correct; Gregory's work is dominated by miracles. But as illustrations of the state of medicine in the middle ages such miracle tales are inaccurate.

They represent the official public attitude of religious leaders, many of whom in actual practice relied on physicians and human medicine. We have already noted the fact that Pope Gregory the Great, author of a popular collection of miracle tales, had faith in the diagnoses and prescriptions of physicians. We must, therefore, look deeper than the miraculous healings in the pages of Gregory of Tours if we would have a true picture of Merovingian medical practice. The most minute and casual references to non-religious medicine must be given as careful attention as the vivid tales of saintly intercession.

So far as supernatural healing is concerned, Gregory furnishes a vivid and detailed picture. Not only in his much quoted *History of the Franks*, but in four other works (*The Miracles of St. Martin, The Glories of the Blessed Martyrs, The Glories of the Confessors*, and *The Passion and Virtues and Glories of St. Julian*) there are valuable fragments of medical information.[105] Inasmuch as Gregory was a prominent bishop and the head of the religious establishments at one of the greatest of Christian shrines, his account of disease and its treatment was completely dominated by the concept of divine intervention. He believed that sickness was the result of human wickedness or divine vengeance; therefore acts of penitence or faith, through the medium of some saint or saint's relics, were the most effective remedy. He constantly lauded the miraculous powers of his own local saint, Martin of Tours. He himself, so he wrote, was cured of headache and stomach trouble by touching the affected member with a portion of the veil with which St. Martin's tomb was covered. Others were healed of sores and hemorrhages by the same means. Gregory also relied implicitly on a sacred potion which contained dust from the sepulchre of St. Martin. His blind faith in this as a cure-all may be illustrated by a passage which reads more like a sacred rhapsody than a medical description:

Oh infallible theriac, Oh ineffable pigment, Oh praiseworthy antidote, Oh purgative which I might even call celestial because it is stronger than the subtle medicines of physicians and it surpasses the sweetness of aromatic spices and goes far beyond the strength of all ointments. It cleanses the bowels like agridium, the lungs like hyssop and purges the head like peretrum.[106]

According to Gregory potions made from sacred herbs which grew near the crypts of the saints could be used with similarly miraculous results. Consecrated oil from St. Martin's or other shrines was equally beneficial. The method of application is illustrated by his tale of the healing of a deaf and dumb man by a hermit. The hermit, he wrote,

grasped the patient's hair with one hand, and drew his head into the window of the cell. There holding the affected man's tongue with his left hand, he took the consecrated oil and poured it into his mouth and on the top of his head saying, ' In the name of my lord Jesus Christ be thine ears unsealed and thy mouth opened.' . . . Then he asked him his name. Whereupon he answered in a loud voice.[107]

Another method was that merely of depositing the patient close to a saint's shrine; a custom very much like the temple-sleep of Greek times and the modern practice at shrines such as Lourdes.[108] One might multiply indefinitely Gregory's accounts of the miraculous healing of the insane, the blind, deaf and dumb, of fevers, paralysis, leprosy, dysentery, stomach trouble, heart trouble, ulcers, gout, colds, sore throat, and aches and pains of various sorts. In some cases even cattle were reported to have been cured of the plague through the miraculous influence of St. Martin.[109]

But these tales are far more convincing as indications of the piety of a Merovingian cleric and his flock than of the absence of real medical practice. It seems probable that Gregory presents more of the miraculous and in more vivid detail than any other known historian. Obviously this material does not present a complete and accurate picture of the medical practice of his age.

Our major problem then is to find evidence of real medical practice even though it be in unsympathetic clerical writings such as his. Such can be found in

the inadvertent references to medical practice in religious writings. This is illustrated by two passages in
a book *Concerning God's Government*, written at
about the year 500 by a priest of Marseille named
Salvian. Salvian wrote almost a century after the
coming of those same Visigoths who, according to
many modern writers, left behind them a trail of
destruction. But he seems to know nothing of any
such cataclysmic effects. On the contrary his work is
filled with references to a still flourishing Roman
civilization, including medical practice, in southern
Gaul. In discussing God's chastisement of his people
Salvian wrote as follows:

Just as the best and most skillful doctors give different
cures for different diseases and heal some by soothing
poultices, employ ruthless surgery for some, but pour healing oil on others, seeking the same good health by different
cures, so also our Lord when he restrains us by harsh blows,
is seeking to cure us by cautery and surgery; when he
favors us with good fortune he is offering us soothing oil
and poultices.[110]

In another equally pious passage he observed that
cattle and flocks are cured by surgery;

When the diseased organs of mules, asses, and swine have
been cauterized they respond to the healing effect of the
fire and at once when the corruption of the infected parts

has been burned away or cut living flesh grows in place of the dead tissue. But we humans are burned and cut yet are not healed by the surgeon's tools or the burning of the cautery.[111]

We can be sure that poultices, soothing oil, and surgery and cautery for both humans and animals were well known to the people of southern France for whom Salvian composed this moral treatise. Salvian's references to surgery, cautery, and medicaments are in keeping with other contemporary records.[112]

There are also indications that medicine was practiced elsewhere. Concerning northern France during the same epoch, Gregory of Tours wrote that Clovis, King of the Franks, had in his palace " a man named Tranquillinus, a doctor well versed in all wisdom, who had won honors in the medical art." But according to Gregory, Tranquillinus admitted that he was " unable to find any suitable medicine " for the king.[113] Therefore he advised calling in a holy man, St. Severinus, by whose spiritual aid the king was eventually healed. In spite of the author's interest in showing the superiority of divine healing, there is in this story valuable information concerning non-religious medicine. The king had a doctor in his palace, probably his private physician, and it is noteworthy that he resorted to divine healing only after having been treated by his doctor. Throughout the Merovingian sources there are similar tales concerning the success of saintly intercession in cases where physicians had failed. Every such account furnishes evidence of the flourishing of non-religious medicine.

Gregory recorded numerous episodes in which the dominating theme of medical failure is accompanied by the revelation that many people resorted to physicians before they called on St. Martin. In fact Gregory himself when afflicted with dysentery and a severe headache went to a physician first. He told of one such experience as follows:

I had suffered so much [from dysentery] that I had no hope of life. The doctor's antidotes were absolutely ineffective. In desperation I called Armentarius the royal physician and said to him: 'You have tried every expedient of your art, and your drugs are of no avail. One thing remains. I shall show you a marvelous cure. Take dust from the sepulchre of St. Martin and make a drink from it.' . . . After taking this drink my pain was eased and I recovered my health.[114]

One of the most unique of Gregory's examples concerns the failure not only of physicians but also of St. Martin. An arch-deacon who was afflicted with cataract, first went from one doctor to another but did not recover his sight even in the smallest degree. . . . [Three months of fasting and prayer at St. Martin's shrine began to restore his sight], but he returned home and called a certain Jew who applied cupping glasses to his shoulders so as to improve his vision. When the blood had been drawn off he relapsed into his former blindness. So he returned to the sacred shrine, but though he remained there a long while he could not regain his eyesight. In my opinion it was denied him because of his sinfulness. . . . Therefore let this be an example to all Christians that when one has been vouchsafed the merit of celestial medicine he should not seek earthly treatment.[115]

Here it will be noted the patient, who was a clergyman, not only began his treatment with physicians but found St. Martin's spiritual power only partly effective and turned to a Jewish healer. This is one of the rare instances in which not even Gregory could find medical success in the intercession of St. Martin.

From the many evidences of this sort in the clerical writings we may be assured of the existence of nonreligious medicine and of a medical profession in the Merovingian times. Let us then, examine the information concerning the various types of practitioners. Apparently medicine was not the well regulated profession of late Roman times nor of early medieval Italy. In most accounts the medical men were designated as *medici*. Gregory used the term constantly in his writings.[116] Most important of all were the royal or court physicians usually called *archiatri*,[117] a title formerly used of Roman imperial physicians. Strange to say the status even of a royal physician was not very high nor secure. One royal physician was a layman of low birth; we are told that " his father had charge of the mills of the church while his brother, cousin, and other kinsmen had been employed in the royal kitchens and bakery." [118] Evidently this self-made doctor prospered in his profession, for twice he was " stripped of all his wealth " by a covetous nobleman. But even worse things could happen. So precarious was the position of a royal physician that he might be executed like a slave at his master's whim. An irate Merovingian queen, on her death-bed, adjured her husband to kill her two physicians because, as she said, " I should yet have hope of life were it not for the potions given by these physicians." The king made, and fulfilled, the requested promise.[119]

But, however badly physicians may have been regarded and treated by Gregory and his contemporaries, they were sometimes reputed to have been very skillful. The words *peritissimus*,[120] *optimus*,[121] and *non ignobiliter instructus* [122] were used of them. At least one of the royal physicians who performed a difficult operation claimed to have been trained in surgery at Constantinople.[123] In this connection we should remember Anthimus, the exiled Greek who served as *archiater* to Theodoric the Ostrogoth, and who was also medical advisor to the Frankish King Theodoric.[124] Occasionally Jews served as royal physicians even though they were generally held in low esteem. Gregory did not even refer to them as *medici*, but merely as Jews.[125] They were however quite common and appear to have had considerable influence.[126] Gregory himself mentions one of them who dared to tell a sick man that St. Martin could not heal him of fever. "No dead man can give medicine to the living," he said. But, adds Gregory, the sick man "despising the words of this old serpent" went on to St. Martin's shrine.[127]

Although there is little detail in Gregory's writings concerning ordinary physicians, their existence is evident from the frequency with which he, Salvian, and other writers mention them. In the early Germanic law codes also we learn that they were numerous enough to necessitate regulation. These same regulations indicate a rather low type of personnel; for instance a doctor was trusted to treat a woman only in the presence of some of her relatives.[128]

There were also practitioners of a lower sort called *harioli* to whom the populace resorted. Gregory mentioned the *rustic* custom of resorting to " sorcery, potions, and the *ligamenta* of the *harioli*.[129] Whether because of the fact that these quack healers were so numerous, or because they competed with St. Martin, Gregory vehemently condemned them, especially in his accounts of the miracles of St. Martin. He displayed quite as much hostility toward the *harioli* as toward the regular physicians, and he vented his spite most bitterly on a miracle-working hermit who claimed to be Christ and who wandered about like a primitive medicine man with a mob of hysterical folk in his train.[130]

Women had little active part in the practice of medicine. A queen such as Radegunde might establish a convent hospice and even go about herself among the sick, bathing them and caring for their sores.[131] There is also some hint of pharmaceutical practice in the account concerning a holy woman named Morigund who healed ulcers by means of prayer, the sign of the cross, and by applying a mixture of saliva and leaves or fruit.[132] In both of these cases, however, the major purpose was spiritual; the medical treatment (if it can be called medical) was of secondary importance. There was of course a great deal of practical medicine performed by midwives and nurses, but France never had a tradition of feminine physicians comparable to that of Trotula and the other women of Salerno.

The evidences cited above concerning the various types of physicians is of considerable importance in the light of the fact that this period is often referred to as the age of clerical or monastic medicine. Most of the *medici, archiatri,* etc. of whom we have glimpses in the pages of Gregory, seem to have been laymen. There are but few cases in which there is indisputable evidence of clerical status, and the hostile attitude displayed by the clergy makes it highly probable that most of the physicians mentioned were laymen trained according to the pagan Roman ideas of medicine. In southern France much of Roman medical practice persisted well into the middle ages. At Marseille, for instance, there is evidence in the fifth and sixth centuries of municipal doctors similar to those of the earlier Roman centuries.[133] In such cities young men were trained and the medical profession perpetuated by lay municipal physicians. Bordeaux also was a Roman medical center. Here in the fourth century members of Ausonius' family studied, taught and practiced medicine.[134] It was Marcellus Empiricus of Bordeaux who compiled a popular handbook of everyday prescriptions.[135] In the sixth century records reveal the names of two physicians of Bordeaux.[136] Lyons and Arles also had doctors.[137] This evidence, scanty as it is, suggests that lay medicine still predominated, and that only in rare cases were the clergy engaging in medical practice. All the known conditions suggest that during the sixth century much of Roman medi- 500-600 cal practice persisted in southern France.

As to the methods used by physicians, we have even less evidence. Inasmuch as clerical writers were chiefly interested in religious healing, they gave no details concerning medical practice. An occasional reference to medicines, cauterizing, surgery, and cupping glasses and sponges for blood-letting is about all.[138] Churchmen made little reference even to the simplest instruments which would be necessary to the surgeon. From archaeological evidences however, we know that surgical instruments of various kinds, and metallic hernia bandages were used.[139]

Practice

Although the churches and monasteries of Merovingian France appear to have lacked professionally
trained physicians, they had institutions in which the
sick were cared for. These were of two distinctly
different types; (1) the monastic infirmary for the
treatment of the resident clergy, and (2) the hospice
or guest house for pilgrims and unfortunates of
various kinds. In accordance with the Benedictine
rule, every monastery provided an infimary, with an
infirmarius in charge, for the care of the ailing
brothers. So far as France is concerned, at Arles as
early as the sixth century Caesarius is said to have
made some such provision for his monks.[140] It is
noteworthy that infirmaries were distinctly monastic
institutions; they did not serve the laity. The secular
clergy inasmuch as they did not ordinarily live a
community life, seem to have had no such establishments.

The secular clergy and the laity are more promi-
nently represented in the so-called "hospitals." In
reality these were hospices (*hospitalia*) or guest
houses (*xenodochia*), in which travellers, pilgrims,
the poor, and unfortunate of all kinds, whether sick
or able bodied, were cared for. Not only the monks,
but also the secular clergy and the laity of Mero-

vingian times took an active part in the founding of such institutions. The Christian ideal of charity made it incumbent on bishops, as well as abbots, to provide for " the stranger within the gates." Kings and queens sometimes contributed funds for this purpose. Of the many monastic, episcopal, and royal hospices and the guest houses in Merovingian France, there are, however, none which were established primarily for medical purposes.[141]

There are two general problems concerning the infirmaries and hospices of Merovingian times: namely the extent to which they provided medical treatment, and the extent to which they were lay institutions. In both cases the answer is " very little." So far as medical practice is concerned, we know that it was subordinate to the practice of brotherly love and Christian charity. Due to the widely prevailing theory that disease was a divine visitation, strictly medical care of the sick by clergymen in clerical institutions was frowned upon. Sufferers could be ministered to and their pain eased, but healing must perforce be left to God, or nature. Thus the infirmary or hospice was by no means a hospital in the modern sense of the word. Treatment was passive, rather than active. The inmates might have special accomodations, special food and perhaps nursing at the hands of clerical attendants who had been given some sort of rudimentary training in medicine. But, at best, medical treatment was rare, and extremely primitive.

Merovingian " hospitals " were very little influenced by the laity. Obviously all monastic infirmaries and hospices were controlled by monks. The hospices established by bishops were likewise manned by clerics, either monastic or secular. As for the royally established hospices, it seems probable that they were clerically managed. In most cases it is clear that the lay founders merely donated the property and income, leaving the administration to the bishop of the diocese and the actual care of the inmates to the lesser clergy. Until the later middle ages, " hospital " service continued to be clerical in spirit and motivated primarily by the non-medical ideal of Christian charity.

Fragmentary though the foregoing information is, it proves without question the existence in France during the Merovingian centuries, of medical men and medical establishments which provided the sick with somewhat more intelligent treatment than saintly relics and superstitious charms. Much of Roman medical practice by laymen continued and in many places the clergy provided for the care of the sick in a systematic fashion. There was also some medical literature. Although there are not many extant manuscripts, the following treatises are known to have been in circulation in various parts of the West during the early middle ages: first, the Latin translations of the most popular works of Hippocrates, Dioscorides, Galen, Oribasius, and Alexander of Tralles; secondly, compilations from classical sources by late Roman writers such as Vindicianus, Theodorus Priscianus, Cassius Felix, Caelius Aurelianus, and Anthimus; and thirdly, miscellaneous compositions in the form of epitomes, letters, and collections of prescriptions.[142]

Among the very small number of French manuscripts of this period which are extant, the Bibliothèque Nationale has two from Chartres dating from the seventh and eighth centuries, and a seventh-eighth century manuscript from Troyes. These contain portions of the *Synopsis* and *Euporiston* of Oribasius, the *Materia Medica* of Dioscorides, the *Therapeutica* of Alexander of Tralles, and other minor treatises, some of which are attributed to Galen.[143] There are also several manuscript fragments containing portions of minor treatises. All in all, practically every important phase of medicine was dealt with. Pathology was represented by works concerning gynecology, wounds, fevers, and a great variety of diseases. In the realm of therapeutics there were treatises concerning blood-letting (flebotomy), purging (clysters), baths, and a mass of materia medica concerned with both compounds (antidotes) and simples (herbs) ; and even *Liber Graduum*. The miscellaneous literature comprised epistles, such as that attributed to Hippocrates concerning the various parts of the human body, also monthly regula, *hermeneumata*, verses (e. g., *de servando medico*), and bits of information concerning food and medical weights and measures.[144] In addition to such material, of which there are definite traces in the contemporary French manuscripts, there undoubtedly existed during pre-Carolingian times many other medical works, similar to those of which we have examples from other regions of the West. The Latin translations of Graeco-Roman medical works, which were produced in considerable numbers in Italy, undoubtedly circulated in France as well as in other trans-Alpine regions. Extant manuscripts give only a faint hint of the sum total of pre-Carolingian medical literature.

more than
we think

Dr. Daremberg, the great nineteenth century French historian of medicine, wrote that in all the realms formerly parts of the Roman empire " there never lacked doctors, medicine, nor medical teaching . . . wherever we turn during the barbarian times we encounter always and everywhere medicine, doctors, and medical schools." [145] So far as medicine and doctors are concerned, we can adopt this optimistic statement as true for Merovingian France, but so far as medical schools are concerned the assertion is unproved and we believe untrue. There were Roman schools for the liberal arts in Italy, and they may have existed in Gaul also during the sixth and seventh centuries, but of medical schools in the modern sense there is no trace whatsoever. Roman medical influences continued in the manuscript literature and in the medical practice, but it seems evident that this was transmitted form the older generation of physicians to their assistants or apprentices in a practical, informal and individual manner. In France, by the sixth century education was practically monopolized by the clergy, and what little medicine was taught, was given as a part of the liberal arts, or in connection with the medical practice of lay physicians, or in the monastic infirmaries. Later, in treating of

79

medical instruction at the cathedral school of Chartres in the tenth and eleventh centuries, we shall find further evidence as to the simple individual character of medical education.[146]

Merovingian medicine, we believe, had two dominant characteristics. Graeco-Roman medical science, which had ceased to progress after the age of Galen persisted, though in a decadent condition. Christian medicine, still in the primitive stage of miraculous healing and nursing of the sick was beginning to advance toward a more intelligent status. During the Carolingian and post-Carolingian ages these two hitherto conflicting influences (Christian and classical) were destined to fuse into a more progressive knowledge and practice.

B. THE CAROLINGIAN AGE

The Carolingian Age and its cultural accompaniments have long been recognized and lauded. In fact the very title renascence, which is often applied to the period, has tended to magnify its achievements at the expense of those of preceding and succeeding centuries. But an examination of Carolingian medicine does not reveal any astonishing advance in medical knowledge or practice. To be sure there is much greater quantity of evidence; this is due to several factors: more was written, and more writings have come down to us. Then, too, northern France was the focal point for the culture of the entire empire including Rhineland Germany and portions of Italy. Therefore, any account of Carolingian medicine is bound to represent many achievements for which France itself was not directly responsible.

The general methods of Carolingian medical practice were the same; as formerly, divine intervention was an accepted theory; and human medicine was still looked upon by many with pious suspicion. The chief difference between the two ages is one of degree; the Carolingian clergy laid much less emphasis on miracles of healing and showed a much more favorable attitude toward human medicine. Nowhere in Carolingian writings can one find such antipathy toward the medical profession as had been shown by Bishop Gregory of Tours.

There is abundant evidence of the increasingly favorable attitude toward medicine and medical men. Among the favorite reference books of clerical students during the Carolingian age were two encyclopedic works, both of which treated of medicine from a secular standpoint. Isidore of Seville's *Etymologies*, which circulated widely during this period, had an entire section devoted to a rational analysis of medicine.[147] Furthermore this subject matter, which was based on Roman medical sources, served as a basis for the medical section of another encyclopedic work. This was compiled in the ninth century by Rabanus Maurus, Abbot of Fulda and Archbishop of Mainz.[148] Thus in the writings of two " dark age " bishops one can trace the continuity of classical medical influences from Roman to Carolingian times. Although neither was French, the works of both were popular in Carolingian France. As a matter of fact, Rabanus was a student of Alcuin, Abbot of St. Martin's of Tours.

Inasmuch as Rabanus took over many of the fundamental medical principles of antiquity his treatment of the subject was free from the bias of miracle healing. This does not mean that his medical ideas were particularly enlightened. Intelligent progress in medicine has often been held back quite as much by blind reliance on classical theories as by stubborn adherence to saintly intercession. Rabanus accepted the misleading classical theory of the humors as the cause of disease. In one passage he wrote as follows:

All diseases arise from the four humors . . . acute diseases which the Greeks call *oxea* arise from blood and bile . . . ancient afflictions which the Greeks call *chronia* arise from phlegm and melancholia.[149]

In a similarly affected classical vein he mentioned various diseases and remedies. His only noticeably religious aberration was a strong tendency to add a religious moral to every description of disease. Thus the various kinds of leprosy are represented as akin to the various kinds of sin; and mandrake because of its many medicinal qualities exemplifies the virtues of the saints.[150] To Rabanus are also attributed treatises of a more practical nature, on anatomy, and a German-Latin glossary of anatomical terms.[151] His writings on medicine are of special importance as examples of the sort of non-religious material which was considered necessary for the education of orthodox Carolingian clerical students.

It is obvious that although Rabanus was one of the most conservative of Carolingian clerics, he was no opponent of medical science. An examination of the medical ideas of other clergymen of the time will further illustrate this tendency. Abbot Lupus of Ferrières, one of the eminent literary clerics of the ninth century, presents an interesting combination of religious and secular attitudes. On one occasion he wrote to a friend saying that a tumor on the groin threatened him with death, but he considered it a blessing in disguise; " it resulted in so many prayers for his recovery that it was a divine benefit." [152] On the other hand he wrote to his nephew recommending a potion to cure headache; if this was ineffective, he suggested calling a doctor.[153] There was no hint of resorting to prayer or any other spiritual method of healing. A century later another abbot, Odo of Cluny, displayed a similar attitude of compromise. On being asked for medicine by two of his monks, he warned them that earthly medicine would do them no good; but nonetheless gave them the requested *medicamenta.*[154]

From abbots such as Odo one might have expected an attitude of pious antipathy toward medicine. On the contrary, during Carolingian times the monastic order seemed to be generally favorable toward medicine and physicians. In the very region which was formerly a stronghold of St. Martin's divine healing, we find clergymen who took pride in medical achievements, especially those of their fellow churchmen. It is a noteworthy fact that in Carolingian and post-Carolingian times this same Loire valley and neighboring centers assumed the leadership in north French culture and medical life. Here, in addition to St. Martin's of Tours, there were monasteries such as Marmoutier, Cormery and Fleury, to say nothing of the episcopal establishments at Tours, Orleans and Chartres. All of these became important medical centers, but during Carolingian times it was the abbots rather than the bishops who played the leading role.

Our most notable example of clerical approval of medicine in this region is Alcuin, monk, abbot and leading scholar of Charles the Great's court. Inasmuch as he was a pillar of religious orthodoxy in Frankland, and also the head of St. Martin's, a popular healing shrine since the days of Gregory of Tours, Alcuin upheld the theory that disease was a divine visitation.[155] But this did not prevent him from holding medical science in high esteem. " It is [he wrote], the science invented for healing and for the tempering and saving of the body." [156] It is evident that this was something more than a mere platitude, for we find him instructing a friend as to the dietary precautions by means of which he might avoid illness while traveling in Italy. He wrote as follows:

Alceun approval of medicine

McKinney missed the point!

Italy is a land of ailments and produces unwholesome foods; wherefor you must watch with the most careful consideration as to what, when, in what manner, and with whom you eat; and especially to avoid drunkenness for it is from the heat of wine that ardent fevers are accustomed to attack those who are not cautious.[157]

It seems probable that Alcuin, like the average educated clergyman, had received some general instruction in medicine. At any rate, he quoted current medical axioms,[158] and wrote with approval concerning those who collected herbs and compounded drugs.

Doctors [he wrote] are accustomed to make a certain kind of medicine from different types of herbs; yet they do not presume to say that they are the creators of herbs or of any other kinds of drugs from the composition of which the health of sick men is regained, but they say they are only the servants in collecting and combining them into one body.[159]

Still more important is the poetical passage in which he described the activities in a Carolingian medical center:

The physicians flock to the Hippocratic halls
This one opens veins while another mixes herbs in a boiler
That one concocts a broth

While another mixes a potion.

But nevertheless, Oh physicians, render thanks for everything

In order that Christ's blessing may attend your labors.[160]

In this case it is interesting to note Alcuin's sane attitude toward religion and medicine. Unlike Gregory, he believed that God worked in cooperation with medical science. The passage also indicates three phases of medicine which were prominent in his day; blood letting, diet and drugs. Of the three, herbal drugs seem to have been the most important. Alcuin mentioned medicinal herbs in several of his letters,[161] and referred in a poem, to "the fields (at Cormery Abbey in Touraine) which bloom with health-giving herbs which the doctors seek for their curative powers."[162] Certain herbs were evidently imported from afar, for he mentioned "a doctor named Basilius who delivered medicaments to you in the mountains en route to Rome."[163]

The prevalence of herb collecting as well as the superstitions connected with the practice are indicated by a contemporary of Alcuin, Bishop Halitgarius of Cambrai. In a treatise, *Concerning Penitence*, he wrote that "It is not permissible when collecting herbs to use incantations or other superstitions unless

McK wants to rescue medicine from the dark ages, but not to explore healing!

with the divine symbol [the sign of the cross] and the Lord's prayer, in order that our Lord may be honored." [164] This passage indicates that the clergy approved of the prevailing medical use of herbal medicines so long as the practice did not encourage the old pagan folk customs which were so persistent during the early middle ages. The popular reliance on what today would be called patent medicines is also illustrated by a rather unusual exhortation found in the writings of Rabanus Maurus. In a manner that is suggestive of the ancient Greek principle of moderation in all things, he gave the warning that " those who drink potions and antidotes continually until satiated are hurt by it." [165]

Even more interesting than the medical reflections of the clerical mind is the attitude of the Carolingian laity. Einhard, Charles the Great's secretary, was one of the keenest observers of the court circles. He was the author of the famous *Life of Charles the Great*, in which, among other things, we find an intimate description of the Emperor's attitude toward medicine. Einhard reported that Charles was very suspicious of physicians. His antipathy was not, however, religious. Like his predecessors he had royal physicians, but he depended on their prescriptions only when it pleased him to do so. According to Einhard:

he relied more on his own judgment than on the advice of the physicians whom he disliked very much because they recommended that he leave off roast meats which he preferred and accustomed himself to those that were boiled.[166]

Einhard's frank explanation of the king's motive and Charles' independent attitude are of less importance to our subject than the fact that the physicians attempted to control the royal diet. Furthermore, Charles was not so irresponsible as might appear from the passage quoted. He seems to have taken considerable pains to preserve his health by dietary regulations. In another passage Einhard reported that

in eating and drinking he was temperate, more particularly so in drinking for he had the greatest of horror of drunkenness in any one . . . the daily service of his table consisted of only four dishes in addition to the roast meat . . . he partook very sparingly of wine and other drinks, rarely taking at meals more than three draughts. In summer after the mid-day repast he would take some fruit and one draught; then . . . nap for two or three hours. . . . [We are also told that] he delighted in natural warm baths, frequently exercising himself in swimming in which he was very skillful, no one being able to outstrip him. It was on account of the warm baths at Aix-la-Chapelle that he built his palace there.[167]

It would be straining the evidence to insist that Charles' diet and recreation were planned according to a scientific regula. However, one cannot help but wonder whether the emperor had a copy of Anthimus' letter or some other such dietary handbook.[168] His sane mode of life is a revelation of the existence during the early medieval times of an intelligent lay attitude toward the problems of health.

Einhard, who wrote of Charles' health, also recorded a few medical details concerning his death. It seems that

for years he was frequently troubled by fevers. . . . While spending the winter [at Aix-la-Chapelle] he had a sharp attack and took to his bed. Immediately, as was his custom, he determined to abstain from food thinking thus to dispel or at least mitigate the fever. But the fever was complicated by an ailment of the side which the Greeks called pleurisy and seven days later he died. . . .[169]

Again in this account physicians are conspicuously lacking. The same absence of any reference to physicians is true of Einhard's descriptions of his own ailments. He wrote as follows:

May my most pious lady deign to learn that I, your servant, have been so afflicted with bodily ills since I came away from Aix that I could hardly get from Maestricht to Valenciennes in ten days. There, so violent a pain in my kidneys and also in my spleen attacked me that I could not accomplish even one mile . . . God is my witness that I write you no untruth in regard to my health, and not only that but also there are certain other ills much more serious which I am suffering, about which I cannot write. . . . If my feebleness of body did not prevent, I should not be sending this letter, but rather coming myself. . . . Because I was not strong enough to ride, I went by water, . . . for an excessive looseness of the bowels and a pain in the kidney followed each other alternately so that there was not a day after I started from Aix that I did not suffer from one or the other trouble. There are likewise other ills which come from that sickness with which I was laid up last year, namely a constant numbness of the right thigh and an almost unendurable pain in my spleen. Afflicted with these sufferings, I am passing a sad life. . . . [170]

If it were not for the fact that we have ample evidence to the contrary, one might infer from these accounts that there were no court physicians or that they were seldom trusted with cases. There are however, numerous references to non-royal physicians. Einhard, for instance, paid tribute to the effectiveness of the physicians in the case of an accident in which a certain nobleman had the lower part of his chest crushed, the right side of his ear torn and his right thigh next to his loins crushed. But . . . the perseverance of the doctors who attended him resulted in a most speedy recovery; twenty days afterwards he went hunting.[171]

The existence of doctors and their methods of treatment of head wounds is revealed likewise in the Carolingian legal codes.[172]

In general the clergy manifested a marked interest in medicine. Far from decrying medical practice Carolingian churchmen often took pride in the achievements of medical men. Walafrid Strabo referred to doctors in a respectful manner.[173] Lupus, Abbot of Ferrières, apparently referred to his own monastic physician in a letter in which he mentioned " our physician who is confident of this ability to heal all infirmities of which anyone has a knowledge." [174] It seems, however, that this physician sometimes failed, for Lupus once wrote to a neighboring abbot, Dido of Sens, asking medical treatment for some of his ailing monks.

Your knowledge of the healing art [he wrote] . . . has become well known to us. . . . Our sons are suffering from bodily ailments, but the doctors whom we have summoned on several occasions have been unable to help

92

them. Trusting in God and your kindness we refer them to you for healing.[175]

Comments such as this are characteristic of the Carolingian and post-Carolingian age. In one respect they present a sharp contrast to the Merovingian picture. There the weight of clerical influence was set solidly against any sort of human medicine. Here the clergy, even monastic leaders, took an active part in medical practice.

Although still in the dim background so far as Carolingian records are concerned, lay physicians, or at least physicians in lay employ, were in evidence.[176] There were as in former times, royal physicians, some of whom may have been clerically trained, or even members of the ecclesiastical order. But in the absence of direct evidence of clerical status it seems justifiable to conclude that doctors serving in a public capacity were laymen. Clerical writers were not prone to leave unmentioned the fact that the incumbent of such a position was one of their order. There is also another uncertain marginal zone, that of lay physicians who became monks. In this category we place Bertharius, a ninth century Frenchman, said to have been of royal lineage, who became a monk and later Abbot of Monte Cassino, where he wrote two treatises on medicine.[177]

As in Merovingian times royal doctors sometimes acquired considerable wealth. One of them, a certain Bishop Everelmus, donated a large amount of property to the church.[178] In the ranks of the purely commercial practitioners were the Jewish physicians who sometimes attained high positions and considerable wealth.[179] Charles the Bald had a Jewish physician who was accused of having poisoned him but seems to have escaped punishment.[180] France, however, had fewer Jewish physicians than other regions. In Salerno, there was a strong Hebrew tradition, and in Moorish Spain Jewish physicians were even more numerous and important.[181]

Of interest in throwing light on the character of physicians and medicine during this period is the program of medical education. Medical education, such as it was, seems to have been far more common than in early modern times. It was a part of the general course of study for all clergymen. Rabanus Maurus in his instructions to churchmen wrote that " the different kinds of medicaments used for varieties of diseases," was one of several subjects concerning which clerics must not be ignorant.[182] The indications are that medical education in the Carolingian realm was broader and, of course, much shallower,

94

than it was in later times. Medicine was not a specialized profession for a few highly trained experts. It was a simple system of empirical treatment, easily learned and easily practiced by any educated man. There is corroboration of Rabanus' statement in a capitulary of Charles the Great's reign, which provided that " all young men are to be sent to learn the medicinal art."[183] This has been interpreted, on one hand, as indicative of a system of universal public education in medicine, and on the contrary as merely a reference to instruction in first aid or nursing. It seems obvious that it referred to all young clerical students and that it was the same sort of rudimentary medical training that was mentioned by Rabanus Maurus. There was no universal system of specialized medical training. For clerics, however, and most educated men were clerics, some sort of medical instruction was practically universal.

Such medical education was closely allied with the liberal arts.[184] In fact, medicine was usually referred to in those days as an art. This relationship was expressed rather quaintly by the sixth century Spanish bishop, Isidore of Seville, whose writings were much used in medieval France. Isidore devoted a section of his *Etymologies* to medical education. In explaining

95

why the art of medicine was not classed with the seven liberal arts, he wrote as follows:

The liberal arts comprise single subjects, whereas medicine involves all. It is necessary for a medical man to know grammar so that he may be able to expound what he reads; also rhetoric, that he may be able to support it with sound arguments; also dialectic so that by the exercise of reason he may investigate the cause of sickness for the purpose of healing; he should also know arithmetic, so as to calculate the times and periods of the day; and geometry so that he may teach what a man should know as to different places; he should know something of music for many things may be done for the sick by this art. Last, let him know astronomy by which he may calculate the stars and changes of seasons; for a physician has said that our bodies are affected by their qualities, and therefore medicine is called the second philosophy. . . . [185]

Silly as much of this seems to us moderns, it does emphasize an ideal that is receiving much attention today, that is, the importance of doctors having a liberal education. Unfortunately, throughout the early middle ages medicine was so completely submerged in the liberal arts that it failed to receive the special attention that it deserved.

Medical education presupposes a medical literature of some kind, and, as we have seen, the early middle ages, not only in Italy but also in France, had a considerable heritage of medical treatises from Graeco-Roman times.[186] In France, the manuscripts of the Carolingian age, as compared with those of the preceding period, contribute an increased quantity of medical literature. There are in existence today five complete manuscripts of medical material,[187] as compared to the three extant manuscripts from the pre-Carolingian age.[188] Furthermore, from the Carolingian period come many medical *fragments*,[189] and a much greater *variety* of material. Particularly noticeable is the large number of brief letter-treatises, usually attributed to Hippocrates, Galen, or some other famous classical physician; these deal with theoretical subjects such as " the four parts of the human body," " the four humors," and " the seven ages of man."

There are also general treatises, bearing titles such as *epitome pereodeoticon, tractatus ysagogus, interrogationes*, or *dogmida*. Of perhaps greater importance are the lengthy compilations of practical remedies; such for example as a *liber medicinalis* comprising 103 chapters, and a *liber medicinalis de omni corpore hominis Terapeutica hoc est collectum ex libris multis philosophorum*, in 110 chapters.

From this period also come the earliest known French manuscripts (in Latin) of Hippocrates' *Aphorisms,* of the *De Morbis* and *De Pulsibus et Urinis* of Alexander of Tralles, and the *Cirurgia Eliodori.* For the first time, also, in French manuscripts, the names of Soranus, Vindicianus, Accius Justus, Quintus Serenus Sammonicus, and Arsenius appear.[190] New titles and new names should not, however, be interpreted as an indication that these works and writers were unknown in the preceding age. For instance, Hippocrates' *Aphorisms* cannot with reason be ruled out of pre-Carolingian France merely by the argument from silence. An actual example will serve to illustrate the danger of such logic. A letter of Accius Justus concerning the human body, conception, and the child embryo, exists in a ninth century manuscript (B. N. 11218), which is the earliest known version. But I find the same treatise, without title and in a fragmentary and almost illegible condition, in another Paris manuscript written in a seventh-eighth century uncial hand.[191] It is reasonable to suppose that a number of such treatises would be revealed if we had the complete manuscripts of the existing fragments from the pre-Carolingian period. In general, the Carolingian manuscripts present the same kind of medical practice as those of the preceding period, but in greater quantity, variety, and detail. Apparently those medical men who delved into the manuscripts that were available, read much the same sort of material as had circulated in the West since the fifth and sixth centuries. And until the eleventh century, medical literature was to continue thus.

The care of the sick and unfortunate, both clerics and laymen, continued as in Merovingian times with little fundamental change.[192] There were two types of institution, the infirmary and the hospice. Hospital service, in the modern sense of the word, is to be found not so much in the hospices (called *hospitalia*), as in the *infirmaria* or *domus infirmarium* of the monasteries. These latter institutions were for the most part monastic, and were intended only for the treatment of the resident clergy, as provided for in Benedictine rule.[193] According to the plan of the ninth century infirmary at St. Gall, it seems that no outsiders, not even novices, were admitted to the monastic infirmary. The novices had a *cella infirmorum* in their own quarters. There was also a separate *domus hospitibus* and a *domus peregrinorum et pauperum*; apparently for the housing of lay visitors, wealthy and poor respectively.[194] It is, however, possible that in case of serious illness lay visitors or novices were taken into the infirmary for medical treatment. There are some evidences of a marked improvement in the medical service of the infirmaries of the Carolingian age. The projected infirmary at St. Gall suggests that medical practice was intelligent and well organized. There are also indications that infirmaries were becoming common among the non-monastic clergy.[195] None of the infirmaries, however, provided anything but nursing, diet, blood-letting, and simple pharmaceutical remedies. The hospices were even less effective in their care of the sick.

So far as hospices and the care of the laity are concerned, the Carolingian records reveal surprisingly few new foundations. Most of the contemporary accounts are concerned with the upkeep or restoration of the older establishments.[196] The most significant trend of the era was the increased effort of the church, with the vigorous cooperation of the government, to universalize this service. We have, for instance, concilar decrees and imperial capitularies prividing for *hospitalia pauperum, xenodochia,* and other types of charity service in monasteries, nunneries, and the houses of the regular canons.[197]

The frequent appearance of the term *hospitalia* and the fact that many of these decrees were semi-governmental ordinances have led some historians to infer that Charles the Great, " declared *hospitals* to be *state* institutions subject to periodical inspection by government officials." [198] This has also been referred to as " the first attempt at the institution of a *secular* care of the sick and poor . . . of royal hospitals under the superintendance of special officials, the *missi dominici.*" [199] Such conclusions must be carefully qualified in order to avoid a double misconception; first, the inference that such institutions were *secularized* during the Carolingian age, and secondly, that they were *hospitals* in the modern sense of the word (i. e., medical centers).

The facts are as follows: the action of Charles the Great and his successors merely gave governmental support to the clergy in their task of expanding the already existing system of hospices. Earlier church councils had gone so far as to decree that the bishops must provide for unfortunates, and that every monastery should have a hospice; similar ordinances were passed in later times. The Carolingian rulers made no more effort to change the clerical status of hospices than of other monastic and cathedral institutions. Under their regime the government joined hands with the church in a more effective manner than before, but merely to assist the clergy in their recognized duty of caring for the unfortunate. Hospices, like schools, were special functions of the church, and Charles the Great gave the clergy effective governmental support in both lines. This was not secularization. There was no fundamental change in the administration or personnel of hospices. As heretofore, these institutions remained under clerical control. It is true that the secular clergy were becoming more active, but there was no hospice service by laymen during this period.

Of greater importance to our present subject is the second possible misconception. Hospices were institutions for Christian charity and not primarily for the medical purposes that are suggested by the modern term "hospital." [201] In the middle ages *hospitalia* was a word more closely associated with hospitality than with medicine. And thus it was with the medieval institutions that bore the name "hospital." They were guest houses and alms houses, not medical clinics. The minor role assigned to medical service in a Carolingian hospice is clearly illustrated by a brief description of the one founded by Bishop Theodulf at Orleans.

Here [he wrote] let the hungry find food, the thirsty drink, the stranger a welcome, the naked clothing, the weary help, the *languid medicine*, and the sad joy . . . [and he added] Let it be open to citizens and strangers.[202]

This brief description is characteristic of the hospices of both Carolingian and Merovingian times.

In conclusion, it may be said of the Carolingian age that the outstanding methods of medical practice were as heretofore blood-letting, diet, and the use of herbal potions of various kinds. Both lay and clerical physicians took part in this sort of medical practice, but without much efficiency in methods of treatment. The most notable improvement over Merovingian times seems to have in the attitude of the clergy toward medicine. They had become actively interested in the improvement of medical conditions. This change was reflected in their increased medical activities. The monks were still more prominent than the secular clergy in caring for the sick. The term "monastic medicine" might well be applied to this aspect of Carolingian medicine. Lay physicians existed, but were not conspicuous. And finally, the Carolingian era did not see an actual rebirth of medicine. In the first place, medical practice had never died out, and secondly,

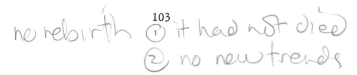

this age is not characterized by any startlingly new elements nor by a sharp upward trend. Charles' greatest contribution to civilization was the centralization and expansion of already existing activities; he was more of an organizer than an innovator.

Hidden away in a footnote in Henry Osborn Taylor's work concerning the medieval mind, is a statement which we believe summarizes the situation so far as Carolingian medical development is concerned. Mr. Taylor writes that

A part of the historian's task is to get rid of epochs and renaissances, Carolingian, twelfth century, or Italian. For such there should be substituted a conception of historical continuity with result properly arising from conditions . . . the Carolingian period did differ in degree from the Merovingian, and the twelfth from the eleventh, but it would be well to eliminate renaissance . . . the word carries more false notions than can be contradicted in a summer's day.[203]

Carrying this theory to its logical conclusion, we are impelled to suggest that it might also be well to eliminate "dark ages" as a characterization of the periods which preceded and succeeded the Carolingian age. It is obvious that the Merovingian age, comprising the three centuries before Charles the Great, saw a steady advance in medical practice in France. Likewise during the tenth and eleventh centuries we shall find that progress was accelerated, especially at Chartres and other north French centers. For the pre-Carolingian and post-Carolingian periods the remark of an eminent French scholar is as pertinent as that of Mr. Taylor for the intervening period. Years ago M. Littré commenting on the tendency of medical historians to omit the early medieval centuries, wrote that " the gap exists in our histories, but not in the facts." [204]

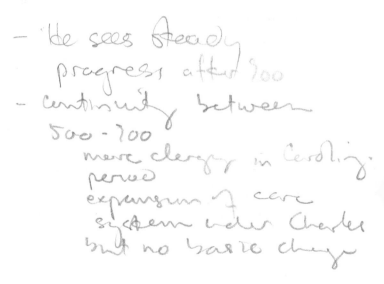

- 'He sees steady progress after 900
- continuity between 500-700
  more clergy in Cerding period
  expansion of care system under Charles but no basic change

MEDICAL PROGRESS AT CHARTRES IN THE TENTH AND ELEVENTH CENTURIES

SPECIALISTS, as well as amateurs, in the study of medieval history are faced with a serious but interesting problem of interpretation. Just as Odysseus was threatened with disaster by both Scylla and Charybdis, so the historian is beset by two dangerous possibilities. On one hand is the traditional tendency to interpret medieval life, and particularly that of the earlier centuries, as barbaric and unprogressive. Equally disastrous, and perhaps more fascinating, is the recent tendency to upset the traditional viewpoint by finding cultural renascence in supposedly dark eras. So far as early medieval medicine is concerned, we believe that he who takes a middle course is likely to avoid serious errors.

We have already given our reasons for rejecting the claims of a Carolingian renascence of medicine. For the ensuing period we feel impelled to steer clear of the contrary hypothesis, which presents a picture of tragic and sudden decline. The popular impression of the post-Carolingian age runs very strongly to anarchy, civil wars, rapine, famine, and constant invasion by savage Norsemen, infidel Moors, and hordes of Hungarians. Many writers and public speakers of our generation continue to perpetuate the modern myth (long ago exploded) concerning a pre-millenial panic which held Western Christendom until the year 1000 transfixed with hysterical terror over the approaching day of judgment.[205]

It is true that France, and particularly the northwestern coastal regions, were afflicted by Norse raids for a little over a half century (about 850 to 910). But the visitations were intermittent, and took toll chiefly of the large and wealthy ecclesiastical centers. So far as the average peasant was concerned, the ravages of local brigands and the wars of neighboring barons were more constant and devastating. But the majority of the population of France lived in peace most of the time. Invasions and wars were not continuous nor universal; although often terribly devastating, they were tempests in teacups. On the whole there was no cessation of settled, civilized life. As in all medieval centuries, epidemics of famine and disease often stalked in the trail of warfare and devastation. With the passing of Charles the Great, the mushroom political unity of his great empire gave way to a decentralized type of government. But France was not plunged into an abyss of darkness, anarchy, and desolation.[208]

For the elucidation of this period, it is our purpose to concentrate attention upon Chartres and certain related centers of north French culture during the tenth and eleventh centuries. The restriction of the field of study to such a small compass serves a two-fold purpose. During this period Chartres was one of the outstanding medical centers of the north, and presents sufficient evidence to make possible a relatively clear picture. By such a " close-up " we are able to gain in completeness of detail what we lose in breadth of view. In the second place it has been asserted, and with justice, that oftentimes an inaccurately favorable view of things medieval is obtained by mobilizing evidences from various regions and centuries into such a complete unity that the sum total appears to be universally characteristic of each of the parts. We shall endeavor to avoid this tendency by devoting our attention almost entirely to medical activities that were related to Chartres.

" The tenth century has a bad name " writes an English medievalist, then proceeds to quote opinions of nineteenth and eleventh century historians respectively to the effect that it was "the wastest place of the human mind" and that "by the year 1000 there was hardly a [worth while] personage, religious or secular in Europe." [207] But the doubting author insists on going back of such returns, and eventually the two gloomy quotations serve as the preface for an illuminating chapter concerning the good things that came out of one of the reputedly darkest of medieval centuries. One of the good things that came out of the tenth century was the cathedral school at Chartres, a then important center about fifty miles south of Paris. During the late ninth and early tenth century, northern France had been in a state of rapid transition. It is probable that unsettled political conditions accentuated the movement by which the old Carolingian centers declined while new and more active cultural centers arose to take their places. One of these was the school of Chartres.

French scholars who write concerning the history of the schools of Chartres, usually present a long and impressive background of early development. Clerval, the most eminent authority, finds schools at Chartres as early as the time of the Gallic Druids, and traces their existence through the Roman, Merovingian, and Carolingian eras. From the time of

Charles the Great on to the climax of Chartres' fame in the twelfth century, he sees no break in continuity.[208] Such a tradition of culture leads one to expect that Chartres might present an unusual example of *medical* continuity. Clerval himself cites evidence from Julius Caesar's *Commentaries* concerning Druid schools " in the region of the Carnutes," and adds significant opinions from two other ancient writers to the effect that the Druids taught medicine.[209] But there is no definite evidence concerning medicine in the early centuries of the history of Chartres. The only evidence is circumstantial; there are constant references to education in the liberal arts, and usually in the medieval era this included the rudiments of medicine. Our earliest definite hint as to medicine at Chartres is the statement of a nineteenth century French scholar to the effect that " a physician of that city, named Amatus, enjoyed a great reputation in the sixth or seventh century." [210] I have been unable to find any supporting evidence for this assertion.

From the pre-Carolingian centuries comes more formidable evidence. There is at the Bibliothèque Nationale in Paris a manuscript (lat. 10233), written in an uncial hand, from the library of the cathedral chapter at Chartres. The manuscript is well known to medical historians because of the fact that it is the oldest and most complete Latin text of Oribasius. It belongs to a French family of Latin manuscripts which were copies of the first translation of the Greek text of Oribasius; a translation doubtless made shortly after his death, in the fifth or sixth century in Italy.[211] The manuscript contains the combined *Synopsis* and *Euporiston*, also Rufus *Concerning Podagra* and several medical fragments.[212]

Quite similar to manuscript 10233 is another Oribasius manuscript (B. N. lat. 9332). This contains not only the Oribasius text but also three books of the *Therapeutica* of Alexander of Tralles, and a *Materia Medica of* Dioscorides.[213] Both manuscripts were brought to Paris, during the French Revolution, from the library of the cathedral chapter at Chartres.[214] The manuscript last mentioned (9332) has been variously dated and located. Leopold Delisle called the script " Lombardic "; [215] and it has been dated by different scholars as seventh, eighth, or ninth century.[216] Several competent paleographers have corroborated my opinion that it is a French manuscript of the pre-Carolingian age, probably from the late eighth century.

So far as I know, every writer on the early history of the schools of Chartres has hailed these two manuscripts as evidence of the early development of medical studies at that place.[217] It is probable that Oribasius, Alexander, Rufus, Dioscorides, and other classical writers were known at Chartres during the pre-Carolingian age, but the manuscripts in question cannot be cited as evidence for the supposition. We have no actual assurance that they originated at Chartres. The fact that they were at Chartres in the eighteenth century does not prove that they had been there continuously for the ten centuries preceding. For one thing the medieval catalogues of Chartres do not list these manuscripts. This of itself is by no means conclusive, for early catalogues were scanty lists, at best, and many manuscripts, particularly those concerning non-religious subjects, would not be mentioned.

But there is evidence which strongly tends to the conclusion that these manuscripts actually originated in another important center; the monastery of St. Benedict at Fleury near Orleans. The comparatively recent science of paleography shows us, more and more, that the internal characteristics of manuscripts are far more important than their present locations, in determining the place of origin. Two of the most eminent of modern paleographers tell me that they see nothing suggestive of a Chartres origin in the style of manuscript 9332; in fact each independently of the other found hints of the style of Fleury. Another expert, who has specialized on the manuscripts of Fleury believes that manuscript 10233 originated at that monastery.[218] Several of its missing folios are now at Berne where many early manuscripts of Fleury turned up after their dispersion following the Huguenot ravages of the sixteenth century. These very folios are bound with two other fragments which are known to have belonged to a book collector who once owned many Fleury manuscripts.[219]

These evidences are of course not conclusive, and since Chartres had the manuscripts in its possession, one may ask; if they originated elsewhere, how did they ever get to Chartres? There are many possible answers to this question. Chartres was closely related to Fleury during the tenth and eleventh centuries. Fleury monks went to Chartres as teachers, abbots, and even bishops. Could they not have carried their manuscripts with them, and could not Fleury have furnished books as well as clergymen to her neighbor? Furthermore, during the Norse invasions manuscripts and other clerical treasures were often taken (as during the World War) to isolated centers for safe keeping. Manuscripts were also borrowed, for the purpose of copying. And sometimes they failed to return. We know of non-medical manuscripts at Chartres which were of unquestioned Fleury origin.[220] So far as our two medical manuscripts are concerned, we suspect that both of them originated at Fleury in pre-Carolingian times and that both were transported to Chartres before the end of the tenth century, perhaps during the period of Norse invasions.[221] Fleury, it might be noted, was ravaged seven times; Chartres, assailed but once, successfully repelled the invaders.

Turning from inference to certainty it can be said that both manuscripts were of pre-Carolingian and French origin. From this we can safely infer that, if not at Chartres, certainly at Fleury or some other French center, there was an active interest in the Latin translations of Greek medical works. In the seventh and eighth centuries, French scholars and physicians were taking advantage of the classical science that had been transmitted to the West during preceding centuries by way of the Italian centers. And interestingly enough, at Chartres in the post-Carolingian age we find traces of this same classical medicine. More concerning this later.

Not until the last quarter of the tenth century is there direct and uncontrovertable evidence of medical activity at Chartres. The absence of information does not, of course, prove the absence of medical activity during the preceding period. On the contrary the advanced type of medicine at Chartres toward the end of the tenth century presupposes a previous development, either of medicine or of a background of education in which medicine might thrive. Cathedral schools had existed at Chartres for centuries, and their program of education in the liberal arts undoubtedly provided elementary training in medicine.[222] But neither Chartres nor the other schools of northern France appear to have placed any particular emphasis on medicine. Fleury, the leading monastic center of this period, does not present a single example of medical practitioners.[223] Rheims likewise, a center as famous for its cathedral school as Fleury and the Loire valley were for monastic education, showed no sign of medical activity until late in the tenth century.

Eventually, it was in the cathedral schools with their traditional emphasis on the liberal arts, that the first outstanding medical progress occurred. At Rheims and at Chartres, men appeared who knew classical medical theory and also had practical experience in medicine. Rheims was the logical place for such a development. During the second half of the tenth century students, both lay and clerical flocked thither not only from all parts of northern France, but from more distant points. Here in a cosmopolitan atmosphere, under the inspiring influence of Master Gerbert, students became enthused over the sciences. As yet, there seems to have been no instruction in medicine as a specialized subject. Richer, one of Gerbert's students, wrote in terms of highest praise concerning his teaching of mathematics and astronomy; he mentioned nothing about medicine.[224] Were it not for other evidences we might infer that Gerbert had no knowledge of, and no interest in the art of healing.

But in his own letters he mentioned the fact that he had studied medicine. To a friend, the bishop of Verdun, who apparently had asked for medical advice, he wrote:

I am willing to consider in detail the special needs of a brother who suffers from gall stones: that is if it be permissible to make use of those things which were provided by our predecessors. Now after you have taken the portion of antidote philanthropos, and observed the instructions for it, it will be your own fault if you turn it to no account by failing to observe the [proper] diet. But do not expect me to handle this matter with the authority of a physician, inasmuch as I have always avoided the practice [of medicine], however much I may have pursued the theory [*scientia*].[225]

It would appear from this letter that Gerbert had a theoretical knowledge of medicine, and that, without assuming a professional responsibility, he was prepared to assist a fellow cleric. On another occasion, he wrote to the archbishop of Treves to say that " if there is anything of the medical art that our efforts can provide, permit us to do it as soon as possible." [226]

Once again he sent the following advice, and possibly medicines as well, to a friend:

Therefore [he wrote], since you are not proficient in the art of healing, and we do not have the materials for remedies, we have taken it upon ourselves to mention those things which the most experienced of physicians consider useful for liver trouble. This ailment you wrongly speak of as *Postuma*, we call it *Apostema* [i. e. abscess]. Now, Celsus Cornelius said that it was called ΥΠΑΤΙΚΟΝ by the Greeks.[227]

This letter is interesting from two standpoints. In

the first place, after promising medical information, it breaks off without anything of practical import. Was the original letter accompanied by a separate sheet of detailed instructions and prescriptions, or can it be that the learned professor totally forgot about such uninteresting things as remedies, once he was engaged in an explanation of the correct form and Greek derivation of the term for liver trouble? The second point of importance in the letter is the characteristic Gerbertian interest in classical books. The citation from Celsus *de Medicina* is exact, a fact which suggests that Gerbert may have had a copy, and used it.

His well known eagerness to acquire copies of ancient books, and the relationship of this hobby to medicine is exemplified in two letters. One of them, written from Bobbio, where he was living in 983, is another curious mixture of friendly helpfulness and all consuming interest in books. He wrote as follows:

If you are getting on well, we rejoice. Your trouble, we make our own, and we ask you to let us know from what you are suffering. Now, the philosopher Demosthenes wrote a book called *Ophthalmicus*, concerning eye troubles and remedies. Let us have the first part of this, if you have it, and also the last part of Cicero's *pro Rege Dejotaro*.[228]

Here again, booklover Gerbert triumphed over Doctor Gerbert; a letter that opened with expressions of sympathy, ended with a request for the loan of two books.

Gerbert's quest for the *Ophthalmicus* did not end with this letter. Five years later he wrote, this time from Rheims (where he was teaching) to Bobbio asking to have a copy made for him.[229] It appears that in 983 Gerbert had been successful in getting an *Ophthalmicus* for the Bobbio library; so later he wrote to Bobbio to get a copy for his library at Rheims. By such devious means were copies of medical, and other treatises, obtained in the early centuries.

In medicine Gerbert was a dilettante. His letters reveal no technical expertness. Even in describing his own ailments he manifested no special interest or knowledge of diagnostic detail.[230] During his later years he wrote the following pitiful, yet ludicrous, description of his many ailments; it is the work of a discouraged old professor, not a physician:

Old age is cutting my last days short. My sides are troubled with pleurisy, my ears ring, my eyes water, and my body is troubled with constant torments. This entire year has seen me confined to my bed with ailments, and now every other day, recurring illness puts me back again when I have just gotten up.[231]

In summary, Gerbert's medical letters reveal the same sort of amateur pharmaceutical practice that we have noted as characteristic of the medically trained clergyman of the early middle ages. But they also reveal a second, and a very different trait: medical book learning. Gerbert had the usual empirical knowledge which made it possible for the well trained cleric to prescribe for his less fortunate friends, but he also had a pronounced academic attitude toward medicine. He knew classical treatises on medical subjects but more often treated them as literature rather than as handbooks of medicine. This separation of medical practice from the book knowledge that was available in classical treatises was, we believe, characteristic of most medieval physicians. Nowhere is it better exemplified than in Gerbert.

In emphasizing the importance of acquiring books, Gerbert did a great service for his age. But by a strange trick of fate not one complete manuscript of the collection he made has survived. There is less extant medical literature from Rheims than from any other major center of tenth century culture. The only known remnant is a ninth century manuscript, now

120

at Paris (B. N. 9347) which contains a paltry seven folios of medical material comprising a portion of the *Liber Medicinalis* of Quintus Serenus Samonicus.[232]

Although Gerbert himself did not rank high as a physician, his school at Rheims had a part in the education of the three outstanding medical men who gave Chartres its reputation. One of them, Heribrand, was a teacher of medicine, another, Richer, an historian and medical academician somewhat similar to Gerbert; the third, Bishop Fulbert, was an amateur practitioner who, like Gerbert, avoided the profession of medicine, but knew how to prescribe and compound remedies. Although all three attended the cathedral school of Rheims during the period of Gerbert's greatest popularity, there is no evidence that he ever taught them medicine. In fact, one of them, Richer, left Rheims to get special medical training at Chartres.

Richer's experience, we believe, exemplifies a universal situation, so far as medical education was concerned during the early middle ages. It was carried on in two ways. The rudiments were taught to young clerics and laymen as a part of the liberal arts program. The relatively small number who went beyond this preliminary stage, were trained individually by lay or clerical physicians. Thus we find that there was no specific medical course at a school such as Rheims. If a young man chose to perfect himself in the medical art, he must find an expert. Gerbert was not a medical expert, nor was there any such at Rheims. Therefore Richer went to Chartres, where another of Gerbert's students, Heribrand, had made a reputation as a specialist in medicine. At this point we turn to Richer for information concerning his studies at Rheims and Chartres. In his *History* (IV, 50) he wrote as follows:

. . . While I was living in the city of Rheims constantly and deeply engaged in the study of the liberal arts and anxious to master the *Logica* of Hippocrates of Cos, I one day chanced to meet a horseman from Chartres. When I questioned him . . . he replied that he was a messenger from Heribrand, cleric of Chartres, and that he wished to speak with Richer, monk of St. Remi. Recognizing at once the name of a friend, and understanding the reason for the message, I made known to him that I was the one he sought . . . Immediately he produced his letter. It was an urgent invitation to [come and] read the *Aphorisms* with him. I was greatly pleased at the prospect and . . . made my preparations to start for Chartres in company with the horseman. . . . [On arriving] I entered diligently into the study of the *Aphorisms* with Master Heribrand who was a man of great culture and learning. But in this I learned only the prognosis of diseases, and since such a simple knowledge of ailments was not sufficient for my desires I begged him to read [with me] his book entitled *Concerning the Harmony of Hippocrates, Galen, and Soran.* He granted this also, for he was very eminent in his profession, and well informed in pharmacology, pharmacy, botany, and surgery.[233]

This passage has often been quoted or cited as an unusual example of medieval interest in medicine. For our purpose it is even more valuable as corroboration of the many inferences already drawn from more scattered and fragmentary information. Let us therefore examine it closely. In the first place it fits in with the hypothesis that the school of Rheims was more concerned with medicine as one of the liberal arts than as a specialized subject. While at Rheims, Richer "was engaged in the study of the liberal arts," but was anxious to specialize in medicine. Unable to find suitable teachers there, he welcomed the invitation from Heribrand of Chartres. This episode in the passage presents an interesting side light on Richer's procedure. Inasmuch as he was expecting some such message, it is obvious that he had been negotiating with his " friend " Heribrand concerning the possibility of coming to Chartres to study. That is, the move was a carefully considered part of Richer's educational program.

This program is also worthy of analysis. It began with the liberal arts, then proceeded to specialization in medicine by the study of certain work of Hippocrates. At this point Richer's account fails to fit into our general picture of medieval medical education. We have emphasized practice and empiricism as the methods by which physicians were trained. But here we have the very opposite, a young man who began his medical specialization by studying the works of the leader of the logical, or rationalistic, school of classical medicine. Of the three schools of classical medicine known to the middle ages (namely, the logicists, the methodists, and the empiricists) Richer followed the most purely theoretical.[234] But this choice is understandable when we consider the fact that Richer was not a typical physician. He was a medical theorist, with strong classical and historical tendencies. He was more of a humanist than a medical practitioner. In fact, it is doubtful that he ever practiced medicine. He seems to have been the type of man who in our day might enroll in an institute of the history of medicine for the purpose of studying classical medicine.

124

But Richer was thorough and ambitious in his medical studies. On arriving at Chartres he " entered diligently into the study of the *Aphorisms*," which comprised a miscellaneous collection of about 400 brief clinical notes, devoted chiefly to the symptoms of disease. On completing this, he demanded more serious material. It is a bit of a contrast to the traditional concept of the primitiveness of medieval medicine to find a student who considered the *Aphorisms* of Hippocrates insufficient for his needs because they furnished merely " a simple knowledge of ailments " and dealt " only with the prognosis of diseases." But thus it was that he proceeded to a detailed study of remedies.

Nothing definite is known concerning the treatise which Richer read *Concerning the Harmony [Concordia] of Hippocrates, Galen, and Soran.* Sudhoff and Diepgen have identified it with an *Oxea et Chronia Passiones Hippocrates Gallieni et Surani*, of which there are early manuscripts at St. Gall (ms. 752), Berlin (Philipp, ms. 165), and Chartres (ms. 62). Their decision seems to be based on the similarity of names in the titles. But, as I have pointed out in a special study on Richer, this is not conclusive.[235] I am of the opinion that the *Concordia* was an alphabetical compendium somewhat like the thirteenth century *Concordanciae* which have been published by Pagel. It may have been a collection of remedies excerpted from the works of Hippocrates, Galen, and Soran by Heribrand himself.[235] At any rate it must have been a work that dealt with those subjects (other than prognosis) which Richer felt were inadequately treated in the *Aphorisms*. It seems probable that the treatise dealt with the subjects mentioned by Richer, namely pharmacology, pharmacy, botany, and surgery. These subjects, it may be noted, are not contained in the *Oxea et Chronia Passiones:* it treats of diseases, describing briefly the causes, symptoms, and cures for each.[236]

Richer, knowing that Heribrand was "well informed" on the subjects he desired, proceeded with his advanced medical studies. The suggestion is sometimes made that Richer's reference to four distinct fields of medicine proves that medical education had already become highly specialized; after studying prognosis, one took up separately pharmacology, pharmacy, botany, and surgery. This is an impossible interpretation. Richer studied all four subjects together, under the same instructor, and probably from the same book. Furthermore, three of the categories (pharmacology, pharmacy and botany) comprise one general field, that concerned with drugs or medicaments. Botany was the study of herbs, pharmacology the knowledge of the uses of various substances, and pharmacy the compounding of medicines. As we have already noted, a knowledge of drugs was sufficient for the great majority of medical cases. Surgery (including cauterization) was resorted to less frequently. Diet, or regimen, the third type of medical treatment, was much less prominent; it is not mentioned by Richer either in this connection nor in the medical passages scattered through his *History*.[237]

To summarize Richer's medical education, he had a "premedic" foundation of study in the liberal arts. This was followed by two stages of advanced study, first in prognosis, second in methods of treatment chiefly by means of drugs. So far as methods of study are concerned, we must avoid the inference that Richer attended a medical school. He merely read classical and early medieval treatises on medicine under the tutelage of Heribrand, whose chief function was doubtless the explanation of difficult passages. The procedure must have been much like our early American method of training lawyers; a young man "read law" in the office of an experienced barrister. Richer " read medicine " with Heribrand. There is no hint of any training in direct observation of medical cases, or in experimentation.

There is no certainty as to the extent to which Richer pursued his medical studies or practice. A bit of evidence from his own copy of the *History* suggests that he continued to read medical works. At the end of the manuscript, following a series of memoranda for the years 995 and 996, there is a note which reads as follows: " Send me the book concerning medicine and the various kinds of metals which you brought out this year when we were in the library." [238] This appears to have been a request from Richer that the friend (to whom he was sending his manuscript) let him have a medical treatise. By this time (996), he is thought to have finished the writing of his *History*, and was devoting himself once more to the study of medicine.[239]

It is my opinion that Richer never practiced medicine. He was a theorist who loved to read and write about medical subjects. In the *History* there are, in addition to the account already quoted, twenty-five passages containing descriptions of diseases, mortal accidents, and the like.[240] Some of these are extended analyses of internal disorders. The following is one of the more detailed accounts:

At Laon that same spring, on account of the changing weather, which by the nature of things tends to occur, he began to sicken. Being troubled with the ailment which the physicians call colic, he took to his bed. He had intolerable pains on the right side just above his privates. From the navel to the spleen and thence to the left groin and the rectum, he was stricken with violent pains. His intestines and kidneys were also affected; [he had] constant straining; bloody excretions; at times he lost his voice. Meanwhile he became rigid with the chills of fever. [He had] rumbling of the intestines; constant nausea; vain efforts at belching, swelling of the abdomen, and heart burn . . . at sixty-eight years of age he died.[241]

In this, as in most of Richer's cases, there is a noteworthy lack of attention to methods of treatment, and a high percentage of names of diseases. This suggests once more that he was more interested in the academic aspects of pathology than the practical treatment of disease.

Richer's medical vocabulary is of importance as an indication not only of this factor, but also of his flare for the classical in medicine. Practically all of the terms he used are to be found in the classical and late Roman treatises which exist in manuscripts of this period still conserved in the library at Chartres.[242] He employed a total of one hundred and nine medical terms.[248] About one-third of these names are names of diseases; about ten of these show distinctly classical characteristics. Most of them are words of Greek derivation, such as *emorroides, erysipelas, machronasia, synantica, causon, cacocexia.* In his medicine, as in his historical work, Richer was a confirmed classicist.[244] His explanation of disease was based on the classical theory of humors; he made practically no reference to the supernatural in relation to human ailments.[245]

Richer's vocabulary also contains many technical terms which indicate a fair knowledge of internal medicine, at least in its theoretical aspects. He was familiar with names such as *anus, arterium* (probably referring to air passages), *colum, epar, inguen, ileum, pectus, praecordia, splenes, thorax, umbilicus,* and *ypocundria.* He also used certain terms little known today, such as *dinamidia* (meaning pharmacology), and *squibalas* (for intestinal obstructions).[246] The fact that most of Richer's medical terms are to be found in contemporary manuscripts, corroborates our belief that the medical treatises copied during this period were actually used.[247]

Before leaving the subject of Richer's vocabulary we take note of one other item, the terms he used to denote physicians. It is a current belief that during the middle ages, physicians were called *medici*. This terminology we find practically universal to the end of the Carolingian age. But the assertion made by the chief French authority on post-Carolingian medicine, to the effect that there is no example of the word *physicus* until the twelfth century, is untenable.[248] Rabanus Maurus in his ninth century encyclopedia used *physicus* twice in reference to medical men.[249] Richer used *medicus* twice, and *physicus* three times. On two other occasions he employed the term *cirurgicus* for surgeons.[250] All of which goes to suggest that, by the end of the tenth century, some sort of distinction had appeared in the medical profession. The prevailing opinion at present is that there was no specialization in medicine until the twelfth century. But we find numerous evidences which tend to invalidate this hypothesis. A scholar who has made a special study of medieval pharmacy in France, finds that from the ninth century on, physicians were accustomed to leave the preparation of drugs to *herbarii*, a distinct class of assistants who were held in rather low esteem.[251] In Poitou during the tenth and eleventh centuries the term *apothecarius* was common, though it is asserted that it was not used of any specialized class of pharmacists.[252] In general, the evidence concerning technical names, from Richer and other contemporary sources, confirms our belief that many of the medical changes now dated in the twelfth century, were well under way a century or more earlier.

In sharp contrast to Richer is the career of his teacher, Heribrand, who though his superior in medicine, left no literary record. By the strange irony of fate, we have practically no information concerning Heribrand. He was the greatest medical expert at Chartres, and perhaps in northern France, a man who could draw medical students from Gerbert's Rheims. But all that is known of him is what Richer told; namely that he was a clergyman, that he was " very eminent in his profession and well informed in pharmacology, pharmacy, botany, and surgery." [253] French scholars such as Clerval and Dubreuil-Chambardel find only one additional item; namely that " Herbrandus, priest and canon of St. Mary's " died at Chartres in 1028.[254] In the course of two research trips to Chartres, Paris, and other French libraries, I have investigated every possible source for further facts. The total result is the one word " Herbrandus," in a list of names at the end of a charter of the monastery of St. Peter's of Chartres for the year 987.[255] And so we must leave in almost complete obscurity the man who has the distinction of being the only known teacher of medicine in early medieval France.

The third of the medical men of Chartres was prominent as a religious leader and consequently attained great fame. Fulbert presents a phase of medicine quite different from any we have yet noted at Chartres. Somewhat like Gerbert of Rheims, he was an amateur physician who avoided professional practice. But unlike Gerbert and Richer he was no classical academician. Along with Richer and Heribrand, he had studied at Gerbert's school, and was familiar with the classics, but he was neither a student of classical medicine, nor (so far as we know) did he ever teach medicine.[256] Fulbert was an intelligent, but pious churchman whom one might expect to have relied on supernatural methods of healing. For twenty years, from 1006 to 1028, he was bishop of Chartres, and during this time he was known as one of the pillars of French orthodoxy. Nevertheless, there are, among the many medical passages in his writings, no indications of a reliance on divine healing, and very few references to the supernatural in medicine. The only detailed reference, significantly enough, is from a distinctly religious work. It is a hymn written in honor of Pantaleon, one of the patron saints of Christian medicine. The poem was written for the purpose of showing the ultimate superiority of celestial medicine, but in it Fulbert granted to human medicine a real efficacy and paid tribute to the Hippocratic art as second only to that of Christ.

We Christians [he wrote] know that there are two arts of medicine, one concerning earthly things, the other concerning heavenly things; just as they differ in origin, so also each has its own efficacy. Earthly medics, by long experience, learn of the powers of herbs and similar substances, which completely alter the condition of human bodies. Nevertheless, no one has yet appeared so experienced in this art as to escape difficulties in healing, and some absolutely incurable maladies. To this Hippocrates bears witness, that man, the physician, than whom there was none greater; he who was brought down from the sky by Esculapius. But when Christ, the author of heavenly medicine, appeared, he was able to cure diseased people by mere command, and to raise the dead from the sepulchre.[257]

The letters of Fulbert present more convincing evidence as to his attitude toward medicine. Here he speaks plainly without either pious or classical verbiage, and here he shows that to him medicine was not a science, but an art, an amateur avocation. Three passages in Fulbert's correspondence indicate that he had been trained in the fundamentals of medicine and could prescribe and prepare simple pharmaceutical remedies.

Sometime during his episcopate, he wrote to his friend the bishop of Orleans as follows:

Believe me, Father, I have not labored at compounding ointments since I attained the rank of bishop. Nevertheless, what little remains of that given me by a certain physician, I bestow on you, even though I deprive myself. I pray that Christ, the author of health, will make it beneficial to you.[258]

Fulbert's generosity, and his well stocked cabinet of medicines is pictured in greater detail in a letter written to another bishop:

We rejoice, O friend [he wrote], at your health and at the well being of Ebal. . . . We are sending three Galen potions and an equal number of *diatesseron-theriacs*. Their strength and the method of taking or administering them, is easily found in your antidotaries. We are also sending you the wild nard which you requested; although we do not advise one of your age to wear himself out thus with vomiting. Instead, if it is necessary to have relief, it can be done frequently and harmlessly by means of oxymel

135

and radishes. But surely it is better for an elderly man to stimulate sluggish bowels by means of laxative pills. As to the things, almost ninety in number, which we have of our own accord offered, consider them, and all that we have as your own. Farewell.[259]

This letter is most revealing as to the pharmaceutical books and materials that were available to a tenth or eleventh century churchman, even though he was not a practicing physician. Fulbert's suggestion that the bishop consult his antidotaries (and he used the word in the plural) suggests the wide prevalence of such handbooks in cathedral libraries. Few French libraries have complete antidotaries from this early period, but almost every one has manuscripts, medical or non-medical, which contain folios of prescriptions, or marginal notations of remedies for all sorts of diseases.[260]

Fulbert had on hand drugs of various kinds; both compounds, such as theriacs and potions, and simples such as nard and radish. If his final offer to the bishop refers to things pharmaceutical, he had ninety varieties. This is not beyond reason. The antidotaries that have come down to us from his day list hundreds of *antidota, theriaca, unguenta, cathartica, cataplasma, olea, trociscos, epithemia, pulvera, pilluli,* etc.[261] Fulbert's pharmacopeia comprised at

least three of the many Galen compounds that were
known in the early middle ages. The name of the
famous Roman physician was attached to hundreds
of potions, cathartics, and the like. There were also
innumerable theriacs. *Diatesseron* theriacs were four-
fold theriacs; there were also *diatesseron* antidotes
and purgatives. In another letter, as we shall see,
Fulbert referred to a *hiera* potion, another of the
famous types of medieval drug.[262] Fulbert's knowledge of *simples*, or uncompounded medicines, is
even more interesting. Much of the letter quoted
above is concerned with simple remedies for clear-
ing the bowels. He not only recognized the neces-
sity of proper elimination, but made intelligent
distinctions between violent and moderate methods
of relief. Of two possible methods (emetic or purgative) he rejected the emetic as too violent for an
old man, suggesting purgatives. But of these he
advised mild laxative pills, rather than the more
vigorous oximel and radish.

Similarly intelligent methods of treatment appear
in another letter. It seems that Fulbert had his
assistant, Hildegaire, send a remedy to a friend.
With the medicine was the following letter of instructions:

The hiera potion . . . is to be taken with hot water before twilight. That evening you must not eat. At night sprinkle . . . soft salt, to the weight of one scruple, into the potion. After taking it, sit quietly before the fire, avoiding drafts. It will do no harm to lie down for a while, but do not sleep. As soon as you are inclined to have a bowel movement, walk slowly to the *secessum.* Even if you are thirsty, do not drink anything except a little sour wine mixed with hot water, for your stomach must be rested [diluendum] and relieved [relevandum]. . . . Avoid eating until the cathartic ceases to act . . . and then see to it that you do not overeat. Eat nothing that is constipating or excessively salted. . . .[263]

The potion described in this letter was one of the famous *hiera* " bitters " which were much used in the middle ages. In this case it was doubtless sent in powdered form, to be taken dissolved in warm water with a sprinkling of salt. The injunction to moderation in eating suggests that some attention was also given to diet. More definite evidence of Fulbert's interest in this rather neglected phase of medieval medicine is to be found in his hymn in honor of St. Ceraunus. One section of the poem contains the following advice:

Splendid banquets often upset the moderation of one's speech; indulge the stomach, and intoxication will trouble your mind;

138

If you partake sparingly at a feast, you will be both
blamed and praised . . .
If possible then absolutely avoid banquets;
But if this is impossible, take your place cheerfully,
Taste everything cautiously, holding to your dietary
regula.[264]

Among Fulbert's students were several churchmen
who won greater fame than he in medicine. One of
these was the assistant, Hildegaire, who probably did
much of his pharmaceutical work. It was he who
actually wrote the instructions concerning the *hiera*
potion. Whereas Fulbert's medical ability was unmentioned by any of his contemporaries, Hildegaire
was said to have had " the [medical] art of a Hippocrates." [265] Another disciple, Berengar of Tours,
won medical fame in his native city. An admiring
friend wrote to him:

Who does not admire your ability in the art of healing.
You surpass those who are professional physicians. My
only regret is that the world does not know your worth.[266]

The distinction made in this letter between medically minded clergymen and professional physicians
is important. All of the Chartrains considered so
far were of the first mentioned class, clerical amateurs. There were, however, several men of Fulbert's

Chartres who became practicing physicians and won medical fame and wealth in distant regions. At least one of these professional physicians was a layman, though he ended his life in a monastery. According to Ordericus Vitalis, Goisbert of Chartres was " very skilful in the art of medicine and known by many people." [267] After serving as physician to a prominent nobleman for some time he entered the monastery of St. Evroult, where his medical services were much appreciated. Later he travelled a great deal, and wherever he went he was said to have healed many diseased folk, both rich and poor, friends and strangers. Goisbert's talents were employed most effectively for both the reputation and the financial profit of his monastery. He refused to accept anything for his services, but invited his patients to show their gratitude by giving donations to St. Evroult. Little wonder that he was allowed to travel far and wide. He finally resumed service with his former noble patron and visited England where he treated many of the ruling class of Norman nobles, incidentally winning great fame and ample gifts for his monastery.

Another of the students of the school of Chartres attained even greater fame than Goisbert. He was

Ralph the Clerk, nicknamed Malecorona. Although Ralph eventually took to the monastic life, in his younger days he was a secularly minded nobleman, who studied the liberal arts and had preliminary training in medicine at Chartres, where he became a member of the cathedral chapter.[268] But Chartres cannot claim the credit of having taught him all that he knew of medicine. He travelled widely, even to Salerno in Italy. To be sure when he returned to France it was reported that he learned nothing in Salerno, having found no one there who was his equal in medicine save one very wise woman, the legendary Trotula according to some scholars.[269] The claim that the French-trained Ralph knew more than the Salernitans is little more than an indication that the French were becoming conscious, and also jealous of the expanding medical fame of Salerno. Half a century earlier Richer related an incident of strikingly similar trend, the medical triumph of a French bishop over a Salernitan physician who was his rival at the French court.[270] As for Ralph, after winning a reputation for marvelous cures, he became a monk of Marmoutier. To him is sometimes attributed the remarkable progress of medicine at that monastery in the late eleventh century. Like

141

Goisbert, he contributed his best years and finest talents to monastic medicine.[271]

general 11th century trends

In the careers of these two Chartrains there is interesting information concerning the trend of eleventh century medicine in northern France. In the first place, they travelled widely, rounding out their early training by study and practice in distant regions. Secondly, although cathedral schools and lay influences were prominent in their education, the chief beneficiary of their practice was the monastic order. Much of the high reputation of monastic medicine is attributable to the far sightedness of the monasteries in appropriating physicians such as Goisbert and Ralph and encouraging them to practice medicine for the benefit of humanity and the glory of monasticism.

After Fulbert's day, Chartres continued to produce physicians of ability and renown. Without attempting to enumerate all of them, we may mention a few of the most outstanding. The signatures of " Guiszo, physician," and " John, physician " appear in a charter of the year 1046 in positions of such importance that we can be sure they were men of high rank, probably private physicians to the members of the nobility, after whose names theirs appear.[272] To the best of our knowledge John was a monk who studied at Chartres and then became physician to various noble families, including the count of Anjou.[273] He finally served as physician to King Henry I of France. His chief fame came from the fact that he lost an important case (no less a personage than his royal master), without losing his own reputation or life. As reported by two contemporary chroniclers this was due to the fact that the king had disobeyed his orders and taken a drink of water immediately after a purgative. As told by Ordericus Vitalis, the king,

following his own desire rather than the orders of the archiater . . . after the medicine had begun to react vigorously on his inwards causing him intense pain, secretly demanded a drink of water from the chamberlain. Without the physician knowing it he drank before the purgative had taken effect. O the pity of it. On the next day he died.[274]

From this brief record of the case it looks as though the physician may have been at fault in giving an overdose of purgative. Purging was often carried to excess. Emperor Otto II, in 983, as related by Richer,

in his eagerness for relief [from constipation] took four drachms of aloes; his bowels were upset, diarrhea followed, and the constant flux brought on hemorrhoids, from which blood flowed constantly, and in a few days he died.[275]

Fortunately the fatal responsibility was placed upon the royal patient; a far cry, this, from Merovingian days. As for John, he escaped with a nickname, " the deaf," to remind him of his failure to detect the king's violation of orders in time to avert fatal results.[276]

We can mention only one other eleventh century physician; his career illustrates the wide travels and varied contacts (both lay and clerical) of medical men of this period. Baldwin of Chartres was successively a monk of St. Denis, prior of an Alsatian dependency of St. Denis, and prior of another branch monastery in England. Then for a time he served as royal physician to Edward the Confessor. Sent by that monarch to heal the abbot of St. Edmunds, Baldwin became a permanent resident of the monastery, and finally its abbot. He once visited Rome where he was cordially received by the Pope. After the Norman Conquest of England he turned once more to lay practice. As William the Conqueror's physician he made many trips to Normandy. Because of his medical skill and attractive personality, to his last days his services were much in demand among the higher nobility and clergy.[277]

With Baldwin we leave Chartres and her famous medical sons of the eleventh century. During the twelfth century the literary fame of Chartres came to a glorious climax. In medicine progress was steady, but not spectacular. The century was ushered in by Bishop Ivo, a second Fulbert; bishop and amateur practitioner. Soon thereafter Chartres had a great teacher, William of Conches who expounded Galenic texts, including anatomy. Later in the century Bishop John (from Salisbury), and Peter of Blois manifested considerable interest in medicine.[278] From this time on one finds among the names of members of the cathedral chapter many followed by the title *medicus, apothecarius, phisicus,* or *cirurgicus* [279] In other contemporary records also, there is an increasing number of references to physicians. More noticeable than heretofore are the indications of lay practitioners.[280] The frequency of terms such as *rasator* and *minutor* indicates that barbers were being employed more and more for blood-letting and surgery.[281]

The steady advance of medicine in Chartres is also evident from the increase in medical literature. The manuscripts from these later medieval centuries existing today in the library of Chartres contain, not only copies of the medical treatises used in the early middle ages, but also many additional works. Among these were the current works of Hippocrates, Galen, and other classical writers, also many of the newer Salernitan and Arabic medical treatises, and various types of alphabetical and non-alphabetical compendia.[282] A number of these manuscripts bear the signatures of their donors; among them, Master Pierre Bechebien, a fifteenth century bishop of Chartres who had been royal physician and also dean of the faculty of medicine at Paris.[283] One of the most interesting of the late medieval manuscripts at Chartres is an *Apothecarius Moralis*, from the monastery of St. Peter's. The title indicates the medical mindedness of the fourteenth century monks of Chartres, but it gives no hint of the real character of the book. It was a general handbook of information on all sorts of subjects, ranging from catalogues of books and information concerning the treatment of wounds, to prayers and saintly biographies. Like Rabanus Maurus in the ninth century, the pious compiler attached a moral lesson where possible. But strangest of all is the frontispiece which reveals a quaint effort at combining religion and medicine. In parallel columns are portrayed the activities of an apothecary and the sacraments of baptism and penance.[284] Thus it was that the monastic world rationalized its religion and moralized its medicine.

After the twelfth century the fame of Chartres and her schools was eclipsed by the rising universities with their specialized faculties. As medical education and practice become more completely professionalized, students sought Chartres less and less. The most glorious days of her history were the earlier epoch when culture, and also cathedrals, of a simpler type were in vogue. Modern tourists visit Chartres because of the unaffected charm of her early Gothic sculpture and stained glass. The occasional research professor, likewise, seeks out the library of Chartres to examine manuscripts that are more unusual than splendid. Whatever there is in the medical history of Chartres that is unique also comes from the less glamorous medieval centuries.

The history of medicine at Chartres may be taken as a symbol of the nature and development of human medicine in the early middle ages. It is noteworthy that Chartres has no tradition of supernatural healing; for the earlier centuries there is nothing save the record of liberal arts education. As elsewhere medicine was merely a part of the general training of intelligent churchmen. There were few professional physicians and most medical practice was carried on by amateurs, either lay or clerical. For the post-Carolingian ages Chartres has two remarkable developments, a book knowledge of classical medicine and a sane type of empirical practice. These also are in keeping with the general trend of medical evolution; the early medieval clergy slowly adopted a more favorable attitude toward classical writings and toward human methods of healing.

The fact that Chartres was pre-eminently a priestly rather than a monastic center is also significant. In northern France, the cathedral schools were the most progressive medical centers. To be sure there were monasteries in or near Tours (Marmoutier, St. Juliens, and St. Martins) and others elsewhere (e. g. at Bourgueil, Cormery, Vendôme, Fécamp, and Bec) ; all of them attained medical fame. But their medical development was antedated, and in many ways surpassed, by that of the cathedral schools of Rheims and Chartres. Many a physician whose medical achievements enhanced the reputation of the monastery which he entered in later life, received his early training in a non-monastic center. The reverse process was seldom the case. In the late eleventh century the pioneer work of Rheims and Chartres was amplified by that of other cathedral schools at Paris, Orleans, Tours, Angers, Poitiers, Le Mans, etc. Without overlooking the fact that monastic medicine was more effective in certain respects (notably in hospital service), and that it served humanity and the church with distinction, we believe that the non-monastic clergy were the more progressive. Their wider contacts and more cosmopolitan attitudes made them more responsive to advanced ideas. The average monk, unless he became an abbot or a royal physician, had little opportunity for travel. On the contrary, bishops, priests, and cathedral canons had much contact with the lay world, both at home and abroad. Schools such as that of Gerbert and Fulbert stood at a point of vantage between monastic and lay society. It was this that made them so progressive and so serviceable to a rapidly changing society.

One final point may be noted that was characteristic of Chartres and her neighbors. Their medicine was a combination of classical and empirical elements, comparatively uninfluenced, at least until later times, by neighboring regions. Whatever credit or discredit north French medicine receives should be attributed to native sons and local schools. The north had little contact with Arabic Spain, Salernitan Italy, and Byzantine Constantinople, which were at a higher stage of cultural and medical advancement during the early medieval centuries. Northern France, with little outside influence, struggled slowly from the primitive medicine of barbarism and religious superstition to an intelligent medical science.

It is the story of medical *evolution* that should be paramount in the history of early medieval medicine. Whatever the state of medical science as compared with our own, this age presents a picture of civilization and medical science in the making. The comparative darkness or brightness of early French medicine is a minor factor. Such damning epithets and flattering titles as dark age and renascence tend to obscure rather than to illuminate the real historical picture.

It is therefore with emphasis on the processes of evolution that we would judge the medical history of the early middle ages. This, we believe, can best be accomplished by applying two criteria. First, what progress was made; secondly, what was the prevailing level of medical practice? We began our survey of French medicine with tales chiefly of miraculous healing from the writings of Gregory of

Tours. We have ended it with a medical mosaic derived from the works of such men as Gerbert, Richer, and Fulbert. The contrast in the two pictures makes obvious the conclusion that there was much medical progress during these early centuries.

As to the prevailing level of medical practice no definite answer is possible. The early middle age was a period of transition; no one picture could accurately indicate the status of medicine throughout five centuries. As between the two concepts, medicine as portrayed by Gregory of Tours, and that of Fulbert's day, we unqualifiedly assert that the latter is more nearly the type for the entire early middle ages. Not only in the tenth century, but during most of the preceding centuries, there was much empirical practice and classical theory similar to that pictured in the pages of Gerbert, Richer, and Fulbert. To be sure, there was much superstition, ignorance, and religious intolerance even in the later centuries. But he who seeks to know early medieval medicine will find its true expression, not so much in the shadow of a saint's shrine as in the monastic infirmary and the cathedral school.

NOTES

CHAPTER I

[1] A. Castiglioni, *The Renaissance of Medicine in Italy* (Baltimore, 1934), p. v.

[2] H. Sigerist, "The History of Medicine *and* the History of Science," *Bulletin of the Institute of the History of Medicine,* IV (1936), p. 11.

[3] *Encyclopedia Britannica* (14th ed.), VII, 60 (F. M. Stenton).

[4] C. Stephenson, *Medieval History* (New York, 1935), ch. ix.

[5] Note, for instance, the treatment in E. Lavisse, *Histoire de France* (Paris, 1911), III, part II, 387 ff.; in F. Harrison, *The Meaning of History* (New York, 1908), ch. v; and the emphatically optimistic view given by Dr. J. Walsh, *The Thirteenth the Greatest of Christian Centuries* (New York, 1907).

[6] C. Haskins, *The Renaissance of the Twelfth Century* (Cambridge, 1927).

[7] In Lavisse, *Histoire de France* (Paris, 1911), Luchaire uses the term "La Renaissance Française (Fin du XIe Siècle et Commencement du XIIe)" as a title for Book II of Vol. III, (part II, p. 205 ff.); there is also reference to "la renaissance scolaire" of the eleventh century (p. 198). Whereas Luchaire places the beginning of the "renaissance" in the last quarter of the *eleventh* century, more recent French writers see renaissance characteristics in the late *tenth* century. J. Calmette, *Le Monde féodal* (Paris, 1931), p. 127 deals with "La Renaissance Ottonienne." A. Fliche, *Histoire du Moyen Age* (Paris, 1930), II, 581 ff., applies the "renaissance" concept throughout his treatment of "La Civilization occidentale aux Xe et XIe Siècles. There is a chapter concerning "Le réveil économique," with a section on "La renaissance commerciale"; also a chapter entitled "La Renaissance intellectuelle et artistique." The pages from 597 to 650 are characterized by section headings and frequent references concerning

" renaissance " in various lines of culture. It is evident that French students of the post war generation are being taught that the " renaissance " began during the tenth century.

[8] J. Robinson, *A History of Western Europe* (New York, 1903), p. 87. See also C. Singer, *From Magic to Science* (New York, 1928), p. 61-2, for the assertion that " the lowest degradation of the human intellect was probably about the tenth century."

[9] See below, p. 106 ff. E. Joranson, *The Danegeld in France* (Rock Island, 1923) presents a constructive view of the Norse era.

[10] G. Chesterton, *Chaucer* (New York, 1932), p. 123.

[11] R. Briffault, *Rational Evolution* (New York, 1930), pp. 108-9.

[12] *Encyclopedia Britannica* (eleventh edition), XVIII, 409-11. The ninth-tenth century "was the dark age," writes J. Shotwell (p. 411).

[13] H. Barnes, *The History of Western Civilization* (New York, 1935), I, 737.

[14] *Encyclopedia Britannica* (fourteenth edition), VII, 60 (F. M. Stenton).

[15] H. Sigerist, *Studien und Texte zur frühmittelalterlichen Rezept-literatur* (Studien zur Geschichte der Medizin, Leipzig, 1923, heft 13); J. Joerimann, *Frühmittelalterlich Rezeptarien* (Beiträge der Medizin, Zurich, 1925).

[16] *Medical Life,* XXXIX (1932), p. 30 (by Dr. L. Bragman).

[17] W. Osler, *The Evolution of Modern Medicine* (New Haven, 1921), p. 84 ff.

[18] E. Meyer, *Geschichte der Botanik* (Königsberg, 1854), III, 412-15.

[19] F. Garrison, *An Introduction to the History of Medicine* (Philadelphia, 1914), p. 82 f.

[20] F. Garrison, " Recent Realignment in the History of Medieval Medicine and Science," *American Historical Association Reports* (1920), p. 175.

[21] R. Park, *An Epitome of the History of Medicine* (Philadelphia, 1899), p. 98.

[22] C. Daremberg, *Histoire des Sciences Médicales* (Paris, 1870), I, 254.

[23] A. Castiglioni, *Histoire de la Médecine* (Paris, 1931), p. 243.

[24] L. Thorndike, *A History of Magic and Experimental Science* (New York, 1923), I, 593.

[25] J. Walsh, *Medieval Medicine* (London, 1920), p. 21.

[26] H. Sigerist, "The Medical Literature of the Early Middle Ages," *Bulletin of the Institute of the History of Medicine* (1934), II, 32

[27] E. Greene, *Landmarks of Botanical History* (Washington, 1909), p. 165.

[28] Gregory of Tours, *De Miraculis Sancti Martini,* iv, 36 (P. L., LXXI). ". . . ligamina herbarum atque incantationum verba proferebant; sed nil medicaminis juxta morem conferre poterant periturae. . . . Quae [i. e., filius eius] adveniens ad aegrotam, eamque visitans, amotisque ligaminibus quae stulti indiderant, oleum beati sepulcri ori eius infudit . . . aegra convaluit."

[29] See Gregory's *Miracula Sancti Benedicti,* ch. 26, in *Dialogi,* II (*P. L.,* LXVI, 134); also certain of his letters on spiritual healing, in the *Registrum,* XI, ep. 20, 26; XIII, 45 (*M. G. H., Ep.,* I). It is, however, important to note that in actual practice, Pope Gregory, like Bishop Gregory (see below, p. 67), resorted to physicians for advice and treatment. The pope wrote the following letter to Archbishop Marinianus of Ravenna: ". . . I was greatly shocked to hear that you were suffering from spitting of blood. I have caused careful inquiry to be made of every one of the doctors here who are known to be well informed on the subject, and I have sent you a written statement of what they severally thought and of what they prescribed. Above all things they recommend quiet and silence. I therefore think that you ought . . . to come to me before the summer that I may myself to the utmost of my ability take special care of your health and see to it that you are kept quiet. The physicians say that the summer time is very dangerous for persons suffering from your complaint. Hence I am very much afraid that if, in addition to the unfavorableness of the season, you should be troubled with the cares of your diocese, the disease will become yet more dangerous . . . I do not exhort nor advise, but I strictly

155

charge you not to venture to fast because the physicians say that fasting is very injurious in such cases . . . You must also give up observing the vigils. . . ."

The Latin text of this letter reads as follows: ". . . percussus sum, quia fraternitatem tuam retulerunt de vomitu sanguinis aegrotare. Ex qua re sollicite et singillatim eos quos hic doctos lectione novimus medicos fecimus requiri, et quid singuli senserint quidve dictaverint, sanctitati vestrae scriptum misimus. Qui tamen quietem et silentium prae omnibus dictant; . . . Et ideo videtur mihi ut . . . tua fraternitas ad me ante aestivum tempus debeat venire, ut aegritudinis tuae ego specialiter, in quantum valeo, curam geram, quietem tuam custodiam, quia huic aegritudini aestivum tempus medici vehementer dicunt periculosum. Et valde pertimesco ne si curas aliquas cum adversitate temporis habueris, amplius ex eadem molestia pericliteris . . . Praeterea nec hortor nec ammoneo, sed stricte praecipio ut ieiunare minime praesumas, quia dicunt medici valde huic molestiae esse contrarium nisi forte si grandis sollemnitas exigit . . . A vigiliis quoque temperandum . . ." *Registrum*, XI, 21. See also XIII, 30 for further details of this case; viz., ". . . Et ideo quoniam eruptionem sanguinis patientibus ieiunia medici omnino dicunt esse contraria, his fraternitatem tuam hortamur affatibus, ut reducens ad animum ea quae de aegritudine ipsa est solita sustinere ieiunandi sibi laborem minime imponat. Si autem Deo miserante adeo melioratam se esse ac virtutem suam sufficere posse cognoscit, semel aut bis in ebdomada ieiunare permittimus. Sed illud te prae omnibus studere convenit, ut exasperationem sentire nullo modo debeas, ne aegritudo, quae modo levior et quasi suspensa creditur, per exacerbationem postmodum gravius sentiatur."

[30] Bede, *Historia Ecclesiastica Gentis Anglorum*, III, 2, 9 (Loeb Classical Library, New York, 1920).

[31] *Ibid.*, introduction (by J. E. King), p. xv. See also A. Thompson, *Bede His Life Times and Writings* (Oxford, 1935), which has a chapter (VII) by B. Colgrave on "Bede's Miracle Stories." "There can be no doubt [writes Mr. Colgrave] that Bede himself

sincerely believed that the miracles he described really happened, but his views on the miraculous as set out *in other parts of his writings* [the italics are mine], seem to be hardly in keeping with his work as a hagiographer " (p. 227).

[32] Walafrid Strabo, *Vita Sancti Galli,* II, 6 (*P. L.,* CXIV). " Si quidem et daemonici ibidem, et languentes sunt recreati, aurium claustra reserata, oculorum detersae caligines, mutorum exclusa silentia, paralyticorum eliminata defectio . . ."

[33] Rabanus Maurus, *De Universo,* xviii, 5 (*P. L.,* CXI). " Lippus est quem terrena cupiditas deprimens, mentis oculos ad coelestia contemplanda elevare non sinit."

[34] Walafrid Strabo, *Vita Sancti Galli,* ii. 18. " Et mox oratorium beati Galli confessoris quasi oraturus ingreditur et ante aram ipsius nomini consecratam consistit; quique ad salutem non merebatur audiri, afflictionis quas aliis se irrogaturum juraverat, convenienti satis talione recepit. Nam intestina eius more sartaginis igni superpositae fervere coeperunt et tam dirae viscerum torsiones illum invaserunt ex templo ut sine aliorum adminiculo nequaquam egredi potuisset, sed (quod dicere pudet) egestio naturae turpi impetu prorumpens cum astantes nimio fetore gravaret, sine mora ab ecclesia ejectus, vehiculo quo decedere monasterio posset, sicut rogaverat, est impositus. Sicque immoderato fluore, naturae consuetudine carens vasi in quod egesta defluerent supersedens, eggressus est, et ad vicinum monasterium quod Auga nominatur, cui et tunc praeerat perductus est. Ubi etiam ingravescente languore tantum sibimet famulantibus ob nimium fetorem intolerabilis factus est, ut ei jam pene nullus obsequia impendere solito potuisset. Tali itaque poena multatus, cum hoc factionum suarum praemio post aliquot dies de cloaca corporis spiritum exhalavit."

[35] Thorndike, *op. cit.,* I, 626.

[36] Isidore of Seville, *Etymologiae,* viii, 9 (*P. L.,* LXXXII). " De Magis. Ad haec omnia pertinent et ligaturae exsecrabilium remediorum quae ars medicorum condemnat . . . In quibus omnibus ars demonum est."

[37] Thorndike, *op. cit.,* I, 720; quoting from a ninth-tenth century ms. (Berlin, Phillips, 165, folio 88).

[38] T. O. Cockayne, *Leechdoms Wortcunning and Starcraft of Early England* (Rolls Series, London, 1864).

[39] See Thorndike, *op. cit.*, I, ch. xxv and xxxi, for an excellent resume of late Roman and early medieval remedies, with emphasis on the magical and superstitious elements in Roman medical works, especially Marcellus Empiricus.

[40] Perhaps the best examples of remedies such as are cited in this paragraph can be found in the Anglo-Saxon Leech Book of the tenth century (Cockayne, *op. cit.*, II). That most of this was a heritage from late Roman times, is evident from the presence of similar material in Marcellus Empiricus, Pliny's *Natural History*, and even to a considerable extent in Galen. See Thorndike, *op. cit.*, ch. XXV.

[41] Cato, *De Re Rustica*, clvi; Latin text and translation in the Loeb Classical Library (New York, 1934).

[42] H. Haggard, *The Doctor in History* (New Haven, 1934), p. 267, gives a brief account of this famous case. I am indebted to Professor Shryock for having called my attention to it.

[43] An eleventh century addition to a ninth century ms. of Chartres; ms. 53, folio 88.

[44] From a tenth century ms. of Chartres; ms. 102, folio 88.

[45] See H. Sigerist, *Studien und Texte . . .*, and J. Joerimann, *Frühmittelalterlichen Rezeptliteratur* (cited above, note 15).

[46] Walafrid Strabo, *De Cultura Hortorum*, xvi; English translation by R. S. Lambert, *The Little Garden* (Wembley Hill, 1924), from which the quotations in the text are taken. The Latin text is found in *P. L.*, CXIV, and *M. G. H. Poetae.*, II. . . . " qui ructus nimium convolvit amaros, oris adusque fores, reprimi persaepe videtur." (Citations from *M. G. H.*).

[47] *Ibid.*, xx.

> " Corporis hunc regem turbans si nausia vexet,
> Mox apium lympha tristique bibatur aceto,
> Passio tum celeri cedet devicta medellae."

[48] *Ibid.*, xxv.

> " Cuius amara satis quatientem viscera tussim
> Mensa premit radix."

[49] *Ibid.,* xviii.

> . . . " huius quoddam genus utile vocem
> Raucisonam claro rursus redhibere canori
> Posse putant, eius sucos si fauce voraris
> Ieiuna, quem crebra premens raucedo fatigat."

[50] *Ibid.,* xxi.

> " Praeterea caput infesto si vulnere fractum
> Tabuerit, tum crebra terens imponito sacrae
> Tegmina, vettonicae, statim mirabere vires
> Illius, in solidum fuerit dum clausa cicatrix."

[51] *Ibid.,* xv.

> . . . " necnon si perfidus anguis
> Ingenitis collecta dolis serit ore venena
> Pestifero, caecum per vulnus ad intima mortem
> Corda feram mittens, pistillo lilia praestat
> Commacerare gravi sucosque haurire Falerno.
> Si quod contusum est summo liventis in ore
> Ponatur puncti, tum iam dinoscere vires
> Magnificas huiusce datur medicaminis ultro."

[52] *Ibid.,* x.

> " Si quando infensae quaesita venena novercae
> Petibus inmiscent dapibusve aconita dolosis
> Tristia confundunt, extemplo sumpta salubris
> Potio marrubii suspecta pericula pressat."

[53] Ekkehard, *Casus Sancti Galli,* ch. 2 (*M. G. S.,* II), " Nam uti plurima doctus, cum unguenta quidem facere nosset, leprosus et paraliticos sed et caecos curaverat aliquos."

[54] See below, p. 135.

[55] See R. Steele, *Dies Aegyptiaci* (from *Proc. Roy. Soc. Med.,* 1920, XIII). Mr. Steele suggests (p. 6) that Egyptian Days were considered merely as unlucky days during the early middle ages, and that it was only after the tenth century that blood-letting was prohibited. But, in early mss. such as Paris B. N. lat., 11218 folio 58 and 11219 folio 169, lists of Egyptian Days are preceded by introductions containing passages such as the following: *sanguinem*

noli minuare. The same is true of B. N. 5600, folio 175; B. N. 820, folio 163; B. N. nouv. acq. folio 12; Chartres, 70, folio 135; Rome Vatican, 1783, folio 136 v; Paris B. N., nouv. acq., 356, folio 1 v; B. N. 2825, folio 126 v, 129. In very few mss. of the early centuries which I have examined, have I failed to find definite reference to blood-letting in the treatises on Egyptian Days. See Thorndike, *op. cit.,* I, 695 for references to English mss.

[56] Paris B. N. 11218, folio 34 v; Paris B. N. 11219, folio 32 v; St. Gall, 751, page 360 ff.; and many other early medieval mss. contain brief treatises, or excerpts, *de flebotomia.* See also Bede, *de minutione sanguinis* (Giles' edition, London, 1843), VI, 349-52. Bede does not mention this work in his list of writings (*Ecclesiastical History,* V, ch. 24), and his authorship has been doubted. Note however, his detailed description of a case of unsuccessful blood-letting, in the *Ecclesiastical History,* V, ch. 3.

[57] See below, notes 122, 160.

[58] See below, p. 54 and plan (Plate I).

[59] See below, p. 145.

[60] Paul, *de Vita et Miraculis patrum Emeritensium,* ch. 4. (*P. L.,* LXXX). " Mira subtilitate incisionem subtilissimam subtili cum ferramento fecit atque ipsum infantulum jam putridum membratim compendiatim abstraxit." The passage contains other medical details.

[61] Ekkehard, *Casus Sancti Galli,* ch. 10 (*M. G. S.,* II). " Infans excisus et aruinae porci recens erucae ubi incutescere et involutus."

[62] Note, for instance, in the *Lex Alamannorum Karolina* (*M. G. H., Leges,* Sectio I, III, 117) excerpts such as follows: " Si autem testa transcapulata fuerit ita ut cervella appareat ut medicus cum pinna aut cum fanone cervella tetigit." . . . " Si autem ex ipso plaga cervella exierit sicut solet contingere, ut medicus cum medicamento aut sirico stupavit et postea sanavit " . . . (*sirico* is linen bandage). For military surgery in eleventh-century Scandinavia, see the interesting facts presented by E. Withington, *Medical History* . . . (London, 1894), pp. 221-2.

[63] *Annalista Saxo.* ann. 981 . . . " pro remedio in capite secari " . . . in J. Eckkart, *Corpus Historicum Medii Aevi* (Leipzig, 1723), I, 229.

[64] Walafrid Strabo, *de Cultura Hortorum*, vi, xxi, xxii, xxiv.

[65] See above, note 62, for references to *pinna* and *fanone*; also note 60, for *ferramento*. Rabanus Maurus (*de Universo,* VI, 1) mentioned the *cultrum*. In addition to these surgical instruments, some use may have been made of the many types of classical surgical instruments such as are mentioned in Isidore of Seville's *Etymologiae,* IV, 11. There is also, in a ninth century mss. (Paris, B. N. lat., 11219, folio 36 v), a list of *nomina ferramentorum* comprising fifty or more surgical instruments. On the fly leaf is a notation " pièces fort curieuses et inédites." For surgical bandages, see above note 62.

[66] See below, note 110, on Salvian of Marseille. Note also the reference to " cauterio aut ferro " in the records of the Council of Chalons in 813 (*M. G. Leges,* Sect. III, III, 283).

[67] Thorndike, *op. cit.,* I, 723. I have noted illustrated treatises on cauterization in several late medieval mss. at Paris (B. N.) and Rome (the Vatican, and the Bibliotheca Casanatense).

[68] The text of this treatise, from a ninth century ms. of St. Gall (ms. 762, page 217-60), has been published by V. Rose, *Anecdota Graeca et Graecolatina* (Berlin, 1870), II. 41 ff.

[69] *Ibid.,* II, 44.

[70] *Ibid.,* II, 65. " . . . quoniam prima sanitas hominum in cibis congruis constat, id est si bene adhibiti fuerint, bonam digestionem corporis faciunt, si autem non bene fuerint cocti, gravitatem stomacho et ventri faciunt, etiam et crudos humores generant et acedias, carbunculos et ructus graves faciunt. Exinde etiam fumus in capite ascendit unde scotomaticae vel caligines oculorum graves fieri solent . . . et ita qui se taliter voluerint observare, aliis medicaminibus non indigebunt. Similiter et de potu . . . sed quid plus? ab antiquis dictum est omnia nimia nocent. Nam et de potu " . . .

[71] See my " Dynamidia in Medieval Medical Literature," *Isis,* XXIV (1936), 404.

[72] St. Gall ms. 751, page 395. This epitome, which is very brief, is quoted by V. Rose, *op. cit.,* II, 52, with detailed explanations, and references to other epitomes from later centuries. He also

describes (page 56 ff.) the six mss. of Anthimus; three of them are ninth century mss.; viz., St. Gall 762, Bamberg L. III. 8, and London Sloan 3107 (a copy of a ninth century version).

[73] See below notes 167, 169.

[74] Cassiodorus, *Variae*, VI, 19 (*M. G. H. Auctores Antiqu.* XII). ". . . Nam licet alii subjecto jure serviant, tu rerum dominos studio praestantis observa. Fas est tibi, nos fatigare jejuniis fas est, contra nostrum sentire desiderium, et in locum beneficii dictare, quod nos . . . excruciet . . ."

[75] Note, for instance, the following passage from Rabanus Maurus, *de Universo*, XVIII, 5: " Ad hanc [i. e., medicien] itaque pertinent non ea tantum quae ars eorum exhibet qui proprie medici nominantur, sed etiam *cibus et potus*, tegmen et tegumen; defensio denique omnis atque munitio qua sanum corpus adversus externos ictus casusque servatur." So far as treatises on diet are concerned, there were many in the early middle ages. Most of the extended medical compendia found in early mss. have sections concerning diet, and occasionally one finds brief fragmentary excerpts. There are *liber diaetarum, diaeta Theodori, diaeta Hippocratis per singulos menses,* and other treatises in which the dietetic material is less prominent; e. g., *Epistula Hippocratis ad Maecenatem, Epistula Hippocratis ad Antiochum regem,* and the *dynamidia Hippocratis.* These are, of course, pseudo-Hippocratic works. On this subject, see Sudhoff, " Diaeta Theodori," *Archiv. f. G. d. Medizin,* VIII (1915), 377 ff.; L. MacKinney, " Dynamidia in Medieval Medical Literature," *Isis,* XXIV (1936), 404 ff.; W. Puhlmann, " Die lateinische medizinische Literatur des frühen Mittelalters," *Kyklos,* III (1930), 404 ff.; and for French mss. below, note 144.

[76] Ekkehard, *Casus Sancti Galli,* ch. 10 (*M. G. S.* II). " Medendo autem mira et stupenda frequenter fecerat, quoque quoniam et in aphorismis medicinalibus, speciebus quoque, et antidotis et prognosticis Hippocraticis singulariter erat instructus, ut urina Henrici ducis versute se decipere temptantis apparuit. Qui cum ei urinam mulierculae cuiusdam cameralis pro sua inspiciendam mitteret: Miraculum, ait, nunc et portentum Deus facturus est, quod num-

quam est auditum, ut vir utero pareret. Nam dux iste circa trige-
simum ab hodie diem filium ex utero suo editum ad ubera suspendet.
Erubuit tandem deprehensus ille, viroque Dei, ne se medicare
renueret (nam ad hoc adductus erat) munera misit, feminamque
illam virginem putatam medicis Sanctigallensis supplicem sibi re-
duxit in gratiam. Nam ut prognosticus ille praedixerat, ipsa partum
dederat."

[77] There were available in the West during the early, as well as
during the later middle ages, Latin treatises concerning urines. See
for instance, Paris B. N. lat., 11218 folio 28; Monte Cassino 97
page 26; Monte Cassino 69 page 551; St. Gall 751 pages 324 and
333; St. Gall 759 folio 80. See also W. Puhlmann, *op. cit.,* p. 408
for additional mss.

[78] Ekkehard, *Casus Sancti Galli,* ch. 10. This passage is a continuation of that quoted above, note 76. " Sed et episcopo nostro
Kaminoldo cum fluorem narium diuturnum adductus citissime
sedaret, odorato cruore, variolam morbum die ei tercia praedixit
futurum. Sed pustulas ille die dicta sibi erumpentes cum eum
restringere peteret: Enimvero (ait) facere potero sed nolo, quia
necis tuae reus karrinas tot ferre non potero, quia, si restrinxero,
morti te trado. Pustulasque tandem eruptas ita in brevi sanaverat,
ut nec saltim de una fuerit signabilis. Haec pauca de plurimis,
quae scriptor, pictor, medicus egit."

[79] See below, p. 61 ff.

[80] Cassiodorus, *Variae,* VI, 19 (*M. G. H. Auctores Antiqui.,* XII).
The medical portions of this letter merit quoting in full: " Formula
Comitis Archiatorum. Inter utillimas artes, quas ad sustentandam
humanae fragilitatis indigentiam divina tribuerunt, nulla praestare
videtur aliquid simile quam potest auxiliatrix medicina conferre.
Ipsa enim morbo periclitantibus materna gratia semper assistit, ipsa
contra dolores pro nostra imbecillitate confligit et ibi nos nititur
sublevare, ubi nullae divitiae, nulla potest dignitas subvenire.
Causarum periti palmares habentur, cum negotia defenderint singu-
lorum: sed quanto gloriosus expellere quod mortem videbatur
inferre et salutem periclitanti reddere, de qua coactus fuerat des-

perare. Ars quae in homine plus invenit quam in se ipse cognoscit, periclitantia confirmat, quassata corroborat et futurorum praescia valetudini non cedit, cum se aeger praesenti debilitate turbaverit, amplius intelligens quam videtur, plus credens lectioni quam oculis, ut ab ignorantibus paene praesagium putetur quod ratione colligitur. Huic peritiae deesse judicem nonne humanarum rerum probatur oblivio? Et cum lascivae voluptates recipiant tribunum, haec non meretur habere primarium? Habeant itaque praesulem, quibus nostram committimus sospitatem: Sciant se huic reddere rationem, qui operandam suscipiunt humanam salutem. Non quod ad casum fecerit, sed quod legerit, ars dicatur: alioquin periculis potius exponimur, si vagis voluntatibus subjacemus. Unde si haesitatum fuerit mox quaeratur. Obscura nimis est hominum salus, temperies ex contrariis humoribus constans: ubi quicquid horum excreverit, ad infirmitatem protinus corpus adducit. Hinc est quod sicut aptis cibis valitudo fessa recreatur, sic venenum est, quod incompetenter accipitur. Habeant itaque medici pro incolumitate omnium et post scholas magistrum, vacent libris, delectentur antiquis: nullus justius assidue legit quam qui de humana salute tractaverit. Deponite, medendi artifices, noxias aegrotantium contentiones, ut cum vobis non vultis cedere, inventa vestra invicem videamini dissipare, habetis quem sine invidia interrogare possitis, omnis prudens consilium quaerit. Dum ille magis studiosior agnoscitur, qui cautior frequenti interrogatione monstratur. In ipsis quippe artis huius initiis quaedam sacerdotii genere sacramenta vos consecrant: doctoribus enim vestris promittis odisse nequitiam et amare puritatem. Sic vobis liberum non est sponte delinquere, quibus ante momenta scientiae animas imponitur obligare. Et ideo diligentius exquirite quae curent saucios, corroborent imbecillos: nam videro, quod delictum lapsus excuset, homicidii crimen est in hominis salute peccare. Sed credimus jam ista sufficere, quando facimus qui vos debeat admonere. Quapropter a praesenti tempore comitivae archiatrorum honore te decoramus, ut inter salutis magistros solus habearis eximus, et omnes judicio tuo cedant, qui se ambitu mutuae contentiones excruciant. Esto arbiter artis egregiae, eorumque distingue conflictus, quos judicare solus solebat effectus. In ipsis aegros curas, si contentiones noxias prudenter abscidas. Magnum munus est subditos habere prudentes, et inter illos honorabilem fieri, quos reverentur ceteri. Visitatio tua sospitas sit aegrotantium, refectio debilium, spes certa fessorum. Requirant rudes, quos visitant, aegrotantes, si dolor cessavit, si somnus affuerit. De suo languore te aegrotus interroget, audiatque a te verius, quod ipse patitur. Habetis et vos certe verissimos testes, quos interrogare possitis. Perito quidem archiatro venarum pulsus enuntiat, quid intus natura patiatur; offerentur etiam oculis urinae; ut facilius sit, vocem clamantis non advertere, quam huiusmodi minime signa sentire. Indulge te quoque palatio nostro: habeto fiduciam ingrediendi, quae magnis solet pretiis comparari. Nam licet alii subjecto jure serviant, tu rerum dominos studio praestantis observa. Fas est tibi, nos fatigare jejuniis fas est, contra nostrum sentire desiderium, et in locum benedicii dictare, quod nos ad gaudia salutis excruciet. Talem tibi denique licentiam nostri esse cognoscis, qualem nos habere non probamur in ceteris." This passage is quoted in M. Neuburger, *Geschichte der Medizin* (Stuttgart, 1911), II, part I, 246-7.

[81] Neuburger, *op. cit.*, II, part I, 254.

[82] *Ibid.*, 254-5

[83] See below, p. 68 ff.

[84] Cassiodorus, *Variae,* IV, 41. The letter was addressed " Joanni Archiatro, Theodoricus Rex," and ended as follows: . . . " nihil fieri volumus incivile, cuius quotidianus labor est generali quiete tractare."

[85] Note, for instance, the attitude (and information) in Neuburger, *op. cit.*, II, part I, 254 f.; Daremberg, *op. cit.*, I, 258; and E. Littré, *Etudes sur les Barbares et le Moyen Age* (Paris, 1874), ch. IV. Of greater importance are the opinions of scholars of our own day who are carrying on detailed researches in this field. The work of H. Moerland, *Die Lateinischen Oribasius Übersetzungen* (Oslo, 1932) is well known. Valuable work is also being done by Professor A. Beccaria of Milan on early medieval medical manuscripts, and by Dr. B. Bischoff of Munich on scribes and translators

of the region of Ravenna. Dr. Beccaria informs me that he is publishing a volume on centers of medical study prior to the twelfth century, with a catalogue of 120 medical manuscripts.

[86] *The Rule of St. Benedict,* ch. 36 (*P. L.,* LXVI). "De Infirmis Fratribus. Infirmorum cura ante omnia et super omnia adhibenda est . . . Ergo cura maxima sit abbati ne aliquam negligentiam patiantur. Quibus fratribus infirmis sit cella super se deputata, et servitor timens Deum, et diligens ac sollicitus. Balnearum usus infirmis quotiens expedit offeratur: sanis autem, et maxime juvenibus, tardius concedatur. Sed et carnium essus infirmis omninoque debilibus pro reparatione concedatur."

[87] Cassiodorus, *de Institutione Divinarum Litterarum,* ch. 31 (*P. L.,* LXX). "De Monachis Curam Infirmorum Habentibus . . . Et ideo discite quidem naturas herbarum, commixtionesque specierum sollicita mente tractate: sed non ponatis in herbis spem, non in humanis consiliis sospitatem. Nam quamvis medicina legatur a Domino constituta ipse tamen sanos efficit, qui vitam sine dubitatione concedit; scriptum est enim Omne quod facitis in verbo aut in opere in nomine Domini Jesu facite, gratias agentes Deo et Patri per ipsum [Coloss. iii, 17]. Quod si vobis non fuerit Graecarum litterarum nota facundia, imprimis habetis herbarium Dioscoridis, qui herbas agrorum mirabili proprietate disseruit atque depinxit. Post haec, legite Hippocratem atque Galenum Latina lingua conversos, id est Therapeutica Galeni ad philosophum Glauconem destinata, et anonymum quemdam qui ex diversis auctoribus probatur esse collectus. Deinde Aurelii Caelii de Medicina, et Hippocratis de Herbis et Curis, diversosque alios medendi arte compositos, quos vobis in bibliothecae nostrae sinibus reconditos, Deo auxiliante, dereliqui."

[88] See above, the references given in note 85.

[89] Cockayne, *op. cit.,* I, pp. xli, xlvi ff., lvii, lxxxvii; III, 297 ff. See also H. Berberich, "Das Herbarium Apulei nach einer frühmittelenglischen Fassung," *Anglistische Forschungen* (Heidelberg, 1902), Heft V, for an analysis of the manner in which Anglo-Saxon compilations were put together from various sources.

[90] The following treatises are contained in Monte Cassino ms. 69: (1) Quare ut humor omnis qui in capite residet . . . (2) a collection of remedies, beginning with ad purgationem capitis and ending adversum venena; (3) An antidotary, beginning with Adrianus antidotus; (4) Antiballomena Galieni; (5) a list of synonyms, vocabula herbarum; (6) a fragmentary treatise on weights and measures; (7) a fragment beginning Unguentum Marciatum; (8) a treatise on urines entitled Liber medicinae urinalibus (?) Hermogenis philosophi; (9) Signa effemerorum febrium de urinis et pulsis secundum precepta Dionisii; (10) Capsula Eburnea entitled Epistula prognostica Hippocratis; (11) de febribus acutis; (12) a calendar of Egyptian Days; (13) Pseudo-Hippocratic prognostics; (14) de cibis; and (15) a fragmentary antidotary. The end of the ms. is missing.

[91] J. Clark, *The Abbey of St. Gall* (Cambridge, 1926), p. 123; also below note 93.

[92] G. Becker, *Catalogi Bibliothecarum Antiqui* (Bonn, 1885), p. 53. This catalogue contains 428 entries; entries 423-6 read as follows; " lib. medicinal. artis. volumina II et I parvus; Item libri III medicinalis artis in quaternionibus." It is found in St. Gall ms. 728.

[93] See note 92. Another ninth century list, found in St. Gall ms. 267, comprising 35 volumes given to the library by Abbott Grimaldus, contains a " Medicinalis liber I in quat." A ninth century catalogue of the neighboring monastery of Reichenau, contains 415 entries, of which 8 were medical works. See G. Becker, *op. cit.,* pp. 8-9 (Reichenau), and 54 (St. Gall).

[94] Mss. 750 to 762 at St. Gall today, relate to medicine; also portions of mss. 44, 105, 124, 217, 225, 878, 908; all of which are from the early middle ages. The same is true of mss. 751, 752, 759, 761, and 762. Mss. 753 to 758, and some twenty more mss. date from the later centuries (i. e., XII to XVI). I have examined all of the early medical mss. of St. Gall, and find that the catalogue of mss. by Scherrer is unusually accurate and detailed. There are, however, several minor treatises that do not appear in the catalogue,

Scherrer, *Verzeichniss der Handschriften der Stiftsbibliothek von St. Gallen* (Halle, 1875).

[95] St. Gall ms. 761, eighth-ninth century. Ms. 908, sixth-eighth century, has a *Mulomedicina* in sixth century uncial (folios 277-92).

[96] St. Gall ms. 761 is an insular ms.; and ms. 913 (non-medical, save for a brief section on blood-letting) is probably Anglo-Saxon. Clark, *op. cit.,* p. 299.

[97] See my "Dynamidia in Medieval Medical Literature," *Isis,* XXIV (1936), 406; and V. Rose, *op. cit.,* II, 121 ff., concerning several five-book compendia. St. Gall mss. 751 (folios 182, 262), 752, and 762 have well organized tables of contents; the same is true of Monte Cassino mss. 69 (pp. 261 ff.) and 97 (pp. 33 ff., which is a six-book compendium). Two Paris mss. (B. N. lat. 11218 and 11219), both from the ninth century, illustrate the more haphazard type of compendium. In ms. 11219, however, folios 42 to 171 comprise two "libri medicinales," with tables of contents.

[98] The original manuscript-plan has been published in facsimile. F. Keller, *Bauriss des Klosters St. Gallen vom Jahr 820* (Zurich, 1844). There are numerous published reproductions and sketches based on this facsimile. The best is that of K. Sudhoff, "Aus der Geschichte des Krankenhauswesen . . ." *Archiv f. G. d. Medizin,* XXI (1929), p. 187 ff. See also that by Suppan in *Journ. American Pharmaceutical Assoc.,* IV (1915), 383; and Clark, *op. cit.,* p. 72 ff. So far as is known, the plan represents a building project which was not carried to completion. It does, however, indicate the medical equipment that was considered necessary for a well organized monastic infirmary of the ninth century. See plate I.

[99] In the original plan (see above, note 98, and plate I), the following herbs are listed: lilium, salvia, ruta, rosas, sisimbria, cumino, lubesticum, feniculum, mentha, rosmarino, fena greca, costo, fasiolo, sata regia, gladiola, and pulegium. It is interesting to compare these with the herbs grown on the villas of Charles the Great. According to the capitulary *de villis,* lxx (*R. H. F.,* V, 652): "Volumus quod in horto omnes herbas habeant, id est *lilium,*

rosas, foenigraecum, costum, salviam, rutam, abrotanum, cucumeres, pepones, cucurbitas, *faseolum, cuminum, rosamarinum,* carvum, cicerum Italicum, squillam, *gladiolum,* dragontea, anisum, coloquintidas, solsequium, ameum, silum, lactucas, git, erucam albam, nasturtium, bardanam, *pulegium,* olisatum, petroselinum, apium, *levisticum,* sabinam, anetum, *fanicalum,* intubas, diptamnum, synapi, satureiam, sisimbrium, *mentam,* menastrum, tanaritam, nepetam, febrifugiam, papaver, betas, vulgigina, bismalvas id est alteas, malvas, carrucas, pastinacas, adripias, blitum, ravacaulos, caulos, uniones, britlas, porros, radicis, ascalonicas, cepas, allia, wacentiam, cardones, fabas majores, ipsa maurisica, coriandrum, cerefolium, lacteridas, sclareiam. Et ille hortulanus habeat sub domum suam Jovis-barbam. De arboribus volumus . . ." The marked similarity of these two lists of home-grown herbs, contrasts sharply with contemporary lists of herbs to be purchased at fairs and markets. For instance, at Cambrai the monks of Corbie planned to buy the following imported (?) herbs and spices: " piper, ciminum, gingember, gariofile, cinamomum, galingan, reopontico, costus, spicum, mira, sanguinem draconis, indium, percrum, pomicar, zedoarium, styrax, calaminta," apparment, thyme, gotzumber, clove, sage, and mastick. This list comes from the ninth-tenth century, and is to be found in the appendix of B. Guérard's edition of *Polyptique de l'abbé Irminon* . . . (Paris, 1886), II, 336. From Mainz, about the year 973 comes a briefer list of " spices "; given by A. Schulte, *Geschichte des mittelalterlichen Handels und Verkehrs zwischen Westdeutschland und Italien* (Leipzig, 1900), I, 73. The existence of such lists of medical materials is of great importance; it proves that the people of the West in the early middle ages actually used the substances mentioned in the St. Gall plan and in many of the early herbals. Walafrid Strabo, likewise, in his *Hortulus* wrote in a simple practical fashion concerning many of these same materials. The materia medica of the early middle ages was something more than mechanical scribal copies of classical compendia.

[100] Paulus Diaconus Emeritani, in his *Vita patrum Emeritensium,* ch. 9 (*P. L.,* LXXX, 139), wrote as follows concerning the medical

provisions at the "guest house" of Bishop Masona of Merida. ". . . Xenodochium fabricavit magnisque patrimoniis ditavit, constitutisque ministris vel *medicis* peregrinorum et aegrotantium usibus deservire praecepit, taleque praeceptum dedit, ut cunctae urbis ambitum *medici* indesinenter percurrentes, quemcumque servum seu liberum, Christianum seu Judaeum reperissent aegrotum, ulnis suis gestantes ad xenodochium deferrent, straminibus quoque *lectulis* ibidem praeparatis eumdem infirmum ibidem superponentes, *cibos delicatos* et nitidos eousque praeparantes, quousque cum deo aegroto ipsi salutem pristinam reformarent . . ." It seems probable that this was not an exceptional case, for similar types of medical service are mentioned in Precepta de concedendo Xenodochio, from an early eleventh century section of the *Liber Diurnus Romanorum Pontificum*, quoted by K. Sudhoff, *loc. cit.*, p. 197-8. ". . . concedimus . . . ut in eodem venerabili loco [i. e., xenodochio] *lecta* cum stratis suis tuo studio preparentur, in quibus egros semper suscipias et egenos eisque curam adhibeas et necessaria tribuas, *confectionem oleorum* infirmantibus atque indigentibus annue facias atque prepares, vel omnia quae infirmantium necessitati sunt utilia, *medicos* introducens et curam egris impendens . . . Huius ergo rei *cautelam* habens pre *oculis,* ita te in commissis eiusdem xenodochii utilitatibus vel exhibitionem curarum infirmorum ibidem reiacentium sollertem ac fidelem nec non efficacem exhibere festines . . ." The above evidences, from the sixth and eleventh centuries respectively, suggest that the Xenodochia of the Mediterranean regions during the early medieval centuries had rather effective medical service.

[101] See below, note 160.

[102] C. Singer, "A Modernist's View of Medieval Science," *Annals of Medical History,* I (1917), 435.

CHAPTER II

[103] See L. Paetow, *Guide to the Study of Medieval History* (New York, 1931), pp. 385-8. "Hagiography was the only species of

literature which flourished in the sixth and seventh centuries in Gaul."

[104] Gregory, *Historia Francorum*. The best Latin text is in *Collection de Textes pour servir à l'étude et à l'enseignement de l'Histoire*. (Series I, Paris, 1886 ff.), vols. II and XVI. It is also found in *P. L.*, LXXI. There is an excellent English translation, with an introductory volume of valuable explanations and historical backgrounds; the critical notes accompanying the text are also helpful: O. Dalton, *History of the Franks by Gregory of Tours* (Oxford, 1927).

[105] All four of these are in *P. L.*, LXXI; viz., *de Miraculis Sancti Martini, Liber de Gloria Beatorum Martyrum, Liber de Gloria Confessorum,* and *Liber de Passione Virtutibus et Gloria Sancti Juliani*.

[106] Gregory, *de Miraculis Sancti Martini,* III, 60. " O theriacum inenarrabilem. O pigmentum ineffabile. O antidotum laudabile. O purgatorium, ut ita dicam, caeleste, quod medicorum vincit argutias, aromatum suavitates superat, unguentorumque omnium robora supercrescit! quod mundat ventrem ut agridium, pulmonem ut hyssopus, ipsumque caput purgat ut peretrum."

[107] Gregory, *Historia Francorum,* VI, 6. "At ille apprehensa manu Caesarie, attraxit caput illius in fenestram, assumptoque oleo benedictione sanctificato, tenens manu sinistra linguam eius, ori verticique capitis infudit, dicens: In nomine Domini mei Jesu Christi aperiantur aures tuae, reseretque os tuum virtus illa, quae quondam ab homine surdo et muto noxium ejecit daemonium. Et haec dicens, interrogat nomen. Ille vero clara voce ait: Sic dicor."

[108] Dr. L. Edelstein, of The Johns Hopkins University Institute of the History of Medicine, an authority on ancient Greek medicine, tells me that he has noted in early Greek sources many medical practices that are strikingly similar to those recorded by Gregory. He is of the opinion that there is danger of exaggerating the religious influences in Merovingian medical practice, and feels that the people of Gregory's day were not so different from those of other great civilizations in their earlier stages of development. Dr. R. Shryock of Duke University, author of the recently published

Development of Modern Medicine (Philadelphia, 1936), after reading my manuscript, expressed a similar feeling as to the fundamental primitiveness of the herbal and other medicines employed in both Medieval France and Colonial America. This is, I believe, a reflection of the obvious truth that folk medicine is much the same in all ages. But, I am still much impressed by the fact that religious and folk practices were predominant in the Gregorian record; and much more completely than in early Greek or American times. See R. Livingstone, *The Legacy of Greece* (Oxford, 1923), p. 230 (by Dr. C. Singer) concerning magic and folk medicine in Greece.

[109] It is impracticable to list here the detailed references in Gregory's works. Those in the *History* can be easily checked in the index to Dalton's edition (see " miracles," " medicine," etc.). For Gregory's other works, S. Dill, *Roman Society in Gaul in the Merovingian Age* (London, 1926) is helpful (see index, under " medicine," etc.), I know of no detailed mobilization of the medical passages from all of Gregory's writings, except an unpublished thesis written by one of my students: Fay Dwelle, *Medicine in Merovingian and Carolingian Gaul* (Chapel Hill, University of North Carolina, 1934). This study contains the Latin text of most medical passages, with English translations.

[110] Salvian, *De Gubernatione Dei,* VI, 16 (*M. G. H., Auct. Antiqu.,* I, part I). There is an English translation by E. Sanford, *On the Government of God* (New York, 1930). " Sicut enim optimi ac peritissimi medici dissimilibus morbis curas dispares praestant atque aliis per dulcia medicamina aliis per amara succurrunt, et quosdam curant cauteriorum adustione, quosdam malagmatum placabilitate, aliis adhibent duram ferri prosectionem, aliis blandam infundunt olei lenitatem, et tamen diverssimis licet curis eadem salus quaeritur. . . ."

[111] Salvian, op. cit., VII, 1. " Iumenta ac pecudes sectione curantur et putrefacta mulorum asinorum, porcorum viscera, cum adusta cauteriis fuerint munus medicae adustionis agnoscunt, statimque ubi aut cremata aut desecta fuerit vitiatorum corporum labes, in locum demortuae carnis viva succedit. . . ."

[112] See above, pp. 32, 40 ff.; also Fortunatus, *Carmina*, VI, 12.

[113] *Vita Sancti Severini*, ch. 6 (*M. G. H. Auct. Antiqu.*, I). ". . . homo in domo regis nomine Tranquillinus, doctor et omni sapientia plenus, honores arte medicinae gerebat . . . [He told Clovis] quia nullus ex nobis corporis tuo potest invenire medicinam. . . ."

[114] *De Miraculis Sancti Martini*, II, 1. "Cumque sic ageretur mecum, ut non remansisset spes vitae, sed cuncta deputarentur in funere, nec valeret penitus medici antidotum, quem mors manici-paverat ad perdendum, ego ipse de me desperans, vocavi Armen-tarium archiatrum et dico ei: Omne ingenium artificii tui impendisti, pigmentorum omnium vim jam probasti, sed nihil proficit perituro res saeculi. Unum restat quod faciam, magnam tibi theriacam osten-dam. Pulverem de sacratissimo domni Martini sepulcro exhibe, et exinde mihi facito potionem. Quod si hoc non valuerit, amissa sunt omnia evadendi perfugia! Quo hausto, mox omni dolore sedato, sanitatem recepi." See also III, 34, for an account of the plague . . . "in qua aegritudine nihil medicorum poterat ars valere" . . .

[115] *Historia Francorum*, V, 6. "Leonastes Biturigus archidiaconus, decidentibus cataractis, lumine caruit oculorum. Qui cum per mul-tos medicos ambulans, nihil omnino visionis recipere posset, accessit ad basilicam beati Martini, ubi per duos aut tres menses consistens et jejunans assidue, lumen ut reciperet flagitabat. Adveniente autem festivitate, clarificatis oculis cernere coepit; regressus quoque domum, vocato quodam Judaeo, ventosas quarum beneficio oculis lumen augeret, humeris superponit. Decidente quoque sanguine, rursus in recidivam caecitatem redigitur. Quod cum factum fuisset, rursum ad templum sanctum regressus est. Ibique iterum longo spatio commoratus, lumen recipere non meruit. Quod ei ob peccatum non praestitum reor. . . . Ideo doceat unumquemque Christianum haec causa, ut quando coelestam accipere meruerit medicinam terrena non requirat studia."

[116] See *Historia*, III, 36; VI, 23; VII, 25; VIII, 31; X, 15; also *De Miraculis Sancti Martini*, II, 19; III, 21, 34, 36.

[117] See *Historia*, X, 15; and *De Miraculis Sancti Martini*, II, 1; Fredegarius, *Chronicum*, ch. 27 (*P.L.*, LXXI) also mentions an

archiater. Marilief, " primus medicorum in domo Chilperici regis " (*Historia*, VII, 25), was also of that status (V, 8).

[118] *Historia,* VII, 25. Marilief, " primus medicorum in domo Chilperici regis. . . . Servitium enim patris eius tale fuerat, ut molendina ecclesiastica studeret, fratresque ac consobrini vel reliqui parentes culinis dominicis atque pistrino subjecti erant."

[119] *Ibid.,* V, 36. "Adhuc spes vivendi fuerat si non inter iniquorum medicorum manus interissem; nam potiones ab illis acceptae, mihi vi abstulerunt vitam, et fecerunt me hanc lucem velociter perdere; et ideo, ne inulta mors mea praetereat, quaeso, et cum sacramenti interpositione conjuro, ut cum ab hac luce discessero, statim ipsi gladio trucidentur . . . [The king promised, and] duos medicos qui ei studium adhibuerant gladio feriri praecepit."

[120] *Ibid.,* VIII, 31.

[121] Salvian, *op. cit.,* V, 1.

[122] Walafrid Strabo, *Vita Sancti Galli,* II, 37.

[123] Gregory, *Historia Francorum,* X, 15. Roevalis, the royal physician, told of an operation on a young boy, as follows: " Tunc ego, sicut quondam apud urbem Constantinopolitanam medicos agere conspexeram, incisis testiculis puerum sanum genetrici moestae restitui."

[124] See above, p. 42 ff.

[125] Gregory, *Historia Francorum,* V, 6; *De Miraculis Sancti Martini,* III, 50.

[126] Dill, *op. cit.,* 241.

[127] *De Miraculis Sancti Martini,* III, 50. ". . . obvium habuit Judaeum et eo inquirente quo pergeret respondit: Typum quartanum incurri, et nunc ad basilicam Sancti propero, ut me virtus eius ab infirmitate hac discutiat. Qui ait: Martinus tibi nihil proderit, . . . Non enim poterit mortuus viventibus tribuere medicinam. At ille, despiciens verba serpentis antiqui, abiit quo coeperat."

[128] *Lex Visigothorum,* XI, De Medicis et Aegrotis (*Rec. Hist. Fr.,* IV, 434). Section i is entitled " Ne absentibus propinquis mulierem medicus flebotomare praesumat"; section ii, " Ne medicus custodia retentos visitare praesumat"; section v, " Si de oculis

medicus hyposismata tollat; section vii, " De mercede discipuli. Si quis medicus famulum in doctrina susceperit, pro beneficio suo xii solidos consequatur." The *Lex Salica,* XX, De Vulneribus (*Rec. Hist. Fr.,* IV, 136), has considerable detail concerning wounds but little concerning physicians. There is, however, a reference to " medicatura pro qua solidos viiii componat "; this seems to be a payment for medical attention.

[129] *De Miraculis Sancti Martini,* I, 26. ". . . ut mos rusticorum habet, a sortilegis et ariolis ligamenta ei et potiones deferebant."

[130] *Historia Francorum,* X, 25.

[131] *Vita Radegondis,* ch. 24 (*M. G. H. Auct. Antiqu.,* IV). ". . . per aegrotantes inferens . . ." See K. Sudhoff, " Aus der Geschichte des Krankenhauswesens im früheren Mittelalter," *Archiv f. G. d. Medizin,* XXI (1929), p. 183; also below, note 141, concerning Radegonde's " hospital."

[132] Gregory, *Liber de Gloria Confessorum,* xxiv. " Nam si quis pusulam malam incurrisset et ad eam veniens orationem precebatur, confestimque illa prosternebatur ad supplicandum Dominum et colligens folia cuiuslibet oleris aut pomi, saliva illiniebat faciensque crucem super ulcus imponebat folium; confestimque ita omne venenum evanescebat, ut nihil dignum leti aegrotus ultra perferret."

[133] See L. Barthélemy, *Les Médecins à Marseilles avant et pendant le Moyen Age* (Marseille, 1883), pp. 8-9; and Dalton, *Gregory of Tours' History of the Franks,* I, 416-17.

[134] L. Dubreuil-Chambardel, *Les Médecins dans l'Ouest de la France aux XIe et XIIe siècles* (Paris, 1914), p. 67. H. Waddell, *The Wandering Scholars* (London, 1907), p. 3-4.

[135] Marcellus Empiricus, *De Medicamentis,* edited by M. Niedermann (Leipzig, 1916). Neuburger, *op. cit.,* II, 60, refers to it as " a compendium of the most absurd prescriptions."

[136] Dubreuil-Chambardel, *op. cit.,* p. 67, mentions Silurius and Caesarius.

[137] At Lyons in the fifth and early sixth centuries, a physician named Elpidius won considerable fame; he is said to have been made questor by Theodoric the Ostrogoth, and is also reputed to

have been a deacon of the local church. See E. Wickersheimer, *Dictionnaire Biographique des Médecins en France au Moyen Age* (Paris, 1936), I, 128.; also Dubreuil-Chambardel, *op. cit.*, p. 67, who also mentions a certain Abascantus of Lyons. As for Arles, Caesarius while still a monk of Lerins, was sent thither to study medicine. See below note 140.

[138] Gregory, *Historia Francorum*, V, 6, 36, mentions *ventosa*, and in *De Miracula Sancti Martini*, II, 55, *spongia*; both used in blood-letting. Salvian (above, note 110) refers to instruments for cautery and surgery; and from the year 813 we have a reference to *cauterio* and *ferro*. Records of the Council of Chalons in *M. G. H.*, *Leges*, sectio III, II, part I, 283.

[139] P. Hamonic, *La Chirurgie et la Médecine d'Autrefois* (Paris, 1900) contains illustrations of surgical instruments, some of them from the early centuries. See also *Janus*, VI (1901), 36. Deneffe, "Les Bandages Hernières à l'Epoque Mérovingienne," *Janus*, V (1900), 584, mentions fifth and sixth century hernia bandages found along the Meuse and Somme Rivers.

[140] *Vita Sancti Caesarii*, I, 2, section 15 (*P. L.*, LXVII), "Infirmis vero imprimis consuluit, subvenitque eis, et spatiosissimam deputavit domum in qua sine strepitu aliquo basilicae opus sanctum possint audire, lectos, lectuario, sumptus cum persona, quae obsequi et mederi posset, instituit; locum libertatemque suggerendi captivis et pauperibus non negavit." The Vita also contains (I, i, section 7) the account of Caesarius having been sent from Lerins to Arles for healing during the period when he was a young monk. "Cumque de infirmitate ipsius [i. e., Caesarius] abbas sanctus graviter turbaretur . . . jubet eum imo cogit beatissimus abbas ad civitatem Arelatensem causa recuperandae salutis adduci." See also I, 3, section 29, for a reference to "medicus etiam diaconus Elpidius."

[141] A distinction can be made between institutions (1) primarily for *medical practice,* (2) those primarily for general charity but with some provision for medical treatment (e. g., doctors, sick wards, etc.), and (3) those for general charity and with provision for the care (*cura*) of the sick inmates, but not for the active cure

176

of diseases. The Merovingian (and also the Carolingian) period had none of the first type, that is of real hospitals; there are rare instances of the second; by far the great majority of the hospices were of the third type. It is possible that the monastic infirmary planned for St. Gall (above note 98), with it wards, heated rooms, pharmaceutical dispensary, herb garden, and staff of physicians, might be classed as an example of type (1); but this was an infirmary, not a hospice, and it is not certain that it was ever actually established as planned. Of the second class we have only a few instances. In Visigothic Spain there was a *xenodochium* which provided beds, "delicate foods," and the service of physicians for sick folk (above note 100). Of similar type was that established in Southern France by Bishop Praeiectus of Arvernus. According to the *Passio Praeiecti* ch. 16 (*M. G. S. Merov.,* V, 235), at "Columbarense, xenodochium . . . fabricare curavit; *medicos* vel strenuos viros qui hanc curam gererent ordinavit ita tamen ut semper ibidem xx egrote mederentur, ut stipendia cibi acciperent postquam vero convalescerent, aliis locum curandi darent." I know of no other French *xenodochium* in which there were resident physicians. It is possible that, even though unmentioned in the sources, other hospices had physicians. Such may have been the case at the hospice which Queen Radegonde established at Poitiers; but the only sick care mentioned in the sources is non-medical *nursing.* Therefore, in spite of the emphasis on the care of the sick, this hospice belongs in class (3). Venantius Fortunatus described it as follows in his *Vita Sanctae Radegondis,* ch. 4 (*M. G. Auct. Antiqu.,* IV): " . . . domum instruit quo lectis culte conpositis congregatis egenis feminis, ipsa eas *lavans in termis* morborumque *curans* [i. e., caring for] putredines, virorum capita diluens, ministerium faciens, quos ante lavarat eisdem sua manu miscebat ut fessos de sudore sumpto potio recentaret. Sic . . . palatii domina pauperibus serviebat ancilla . . ." In most of the hospices of Merovingian times there was even less emphasis on the care of the sick. It was the poor, the aged, and unfortunates of all kinds, including the sick, who were ministered to. The *Vita Sanctus Abbatis Eugendi Jurensium Romani,* ch. 21,

177

and the *Vita Ansberti Episcopi Rotomagensi*, ch. 14 (*M. G. S. Merov.*, III and V) make reference to " *infirmus* semper aut valde *senibus*," and " xenodochium *inbecillium* ac *decrepitorum pauperum* . . . Alias quoque duas . . . *pauperum* Christi *debilium* mansiones " (at Fontanelle Monastery). Even the leprosaria, belong in the third class of institutions, devoted primarily to general charity. (See Sudhoff, ". . . Geschichte d. Krankenhauswesens . . ." *loc. cit.*, p. 200-1). For instance, Bishop Agricola of Châlons-sur-Marne built a " Xenodochia leprosarium suburbana " (in the sixth century) ; but it was merely a house in which lepers were lodged, fed, and clothed (Gregory of Tours, *Liber de Gloria Confessorum*, lxxxv-lxxxvi). There is no hint of any medical purpose, except the segregation of the lepers. This is also suggested in the proceedings of the Council of Lyons (583), ch. 6, where it was ordered that the bishops provide the lepers of their communities with " alimenta et necessaria vestimenta," and " illis per alias civitates vagandi licentia denegetur." (*M. G. Leges,* sectio III, I, 154). In similar fashion, two centuries later, a capitulary (Duplex legationis edictum, ch. 36) provided " de leprosis ut se non intermisceant alio populo." (*M. G. Leges,* sectio II, I, 64). It is obvious that such activities were not medical service, but merely a special phase of bishops' general charitable functions. The same sort of non-medical care was provided for the " poor and infirm." According to the regulations of the Council of Orleans (571), ch. 16 (*M. G. Leges,* sectio III, I, part I, 16), " Episcopus *pauperibus* vel *infirmis* qui debilitate faciente non possunt suis manibus laborare, *victum et vestitum* in quantum possebilitas habuerit largiatur." The same function of general Christian charity is evident in the case of the famous *xenodochium* founded at Lyons by King Childebert and his queen in the sixth century. It was to be devoted forever to " the care of the sick " (cura aegrotantium), of pilgrims, and of the poor. (Council of Orleans of the year 549, ch. 15; *M. G. Leges,* sectio III, I, part I, 105). Here, as in numerous other cases, " cura aegrotantium " was not medical treatment, but food, clothing, and shelter, similar to that provided for all unfortunates. Those who were seriously ill were doubtless given some sort of nursing. Of similar character, and therefore properly belonging to class 3, we consider King Childebert's Hôtel Dieu at Paris, King Dagobert's hospice in Paris, and the famous " xenodochium *pauperibus* ac *peregrinis* " founded at Autun in the sixth century by Bishop Syagrius and Queen Brunhilde (Gregory I, *Epistula,* XIII, 11; *M. G. Ep.* I). The same holds true for clerical foundations such as that of Bishop Remigius at Rheims, of St. Nicholas at Nivelles, of the brothers and sisters of St. Victor at Tournai, and the numerous *hospitalia Scotorum* in northern France (Sudhoff, ". . . Geschichte d. Krankenhauswesens . . .", *loc. cit.,* p. 183. See also Gregory of Tours, *Historia,* VI, 45, and his *de Miraculis S. Martini,* II, 27, for references to "hospitalia pauperum"; also *M. G. S. Merov.,* IV, 682; V, 557, 628; and VII, 9, for references to *xenodochia* established by bishops (*Vita Audoini Episcopi Rotomagensis,* II, ch. 24; and *Vita Eligii Episcopi Novimagensis,* I, ch. 17), and by abbots (*Vita Menelei Abbatis Menatensis,* II, 2; and *Vita Leutfredi Abbatis Madriacensis,* ch. 24). In general, it seems probable that most bishops and abbots of Merovingian times had some sort of guest houses in which they dispensed charity to pilgrims, the aged, the infirm, and unfortunates of all kinds. In these institutions there was no real medical treatment, and whatever there was of " care for the sick," was a simple type of nursing. They should not be thought of as hospitals.

[142] On this matter see the opinions of two great French scholars of the nineteenth century: C. Daremberg, *op. cit.,* I, 255, 278; and E. Littré, *op. cit.,* p. 263 ff. See also above, note 95.

[143] Paris B. N. 10233 and 9332 (both from Chartres), and nouv. acq. 1619 (from Troyes). For detailed descriptions of these mss., see below notes 212-13.

[144] Paris B. N. nouv. acq. 203 (seventh-eighth century fragment of 4 pp.) contains the following, though in almost totally illegible condition: f. 1 (unidentifiable material) . . . ydropsa . . . in loca impona frigida . . . vena . . . aqua . . .; (receptaria); f. 2 epistula Acii Justi (concerning the human body, gynecology, etc.) . . . mulier . . . menstrua . . . semen . . . sanguinis . . . semen mascu-

linum . . . dentes . . . xxx in utero . . . nona mense . . .; f. 3
(remedies) . . . ad febres . . .; (fragment on flebotomy); de ponderibus Goronimis . . .; f. 4 ep. ypogratis de naturas humana vel
conceptionem eorum, nunc ex liber Gregorum (?) liber certat . . .
(deals with parts of the body).   In another ms. (B. N. 10318) from
the eighth century are the following: p. 82-95 de balneis (in verse);
p. 112 de servando medico (in verse); p. 196-204 brevis pimentorum qui in domo esse debeant. crocum piper . . . Brevis ciborum (31
chapters on various kinds of foods); p. 204 de ponderibus (title
only); p. 262 ff. de remediis salutaribus Apulei Platoni; p. 266-73
de herbis antiquitas mirataes . . . (with additional sections of the
de remediis and fragments of other materials interspersed; the pages
are badly jumbled and several are out of place).   Another eighth
century ms (B. N. nouv. acq., 1619, f. 206-7) contains remedies ad
morbo regio . . . and a pocio aposmtcis (?).   Although fragmentary
and in very uncertain condition these mss. serve to illustrate the fact
that the pre-Carolingian era had a considerable medical literature
comprising treatises on gynecology, diseases, flebotomy, weights and
measures, baths, diet, herbals and antidotaries.   I have found no
reference to these mss. in standard works such as H. Diels, *Die
Handschriften der Antiken Ärzte* (Berlin, 1905).   Inasmuch as the
B. N. catalogues are entirely inadequate, I have given the contents
in some detail.   Of similar importance are the minor treatises which
appear in the better known mss.   For instance B. N. 9332, f. 251
has Epistula uulter. Provinciae Babiloniae Alexandria regis Romae
salutem.   B. N. 10233, f. 263-79 contains the following: Rufus de
Podagra (31 chapters); Graefadia ex alio auctore ad podagra;
Virtus herbae peonia; Curatio Flegmonis . . . (and other remedies);
de parotidis et inguinibus . . . de masculis . . . de nervis nervorum
. . .; a series of cataplasmata, laxatives, and finally malagma ad
artriticos; the mss. ends (f. 279-80) with an Oribase fragment de
praebidendis passionibus, and de reu ponticu ex alio auctore.   In
British libraries there are many mss. of French origin; among those
from the early centuries which contain medical material, are the
following, which doubtless originated in southern France (possi-

bly in northern Italy). London, Harley 5792(seventh-eighth century), is a ms. that is related to a ms. of Laon; f. 273-6 contain medical prescriptions. Glasgow, Hunter T. 4. 13, is an eighth-ninth century ms. in pre-Carolingian minuscule; so similar in script to Paris B. N. nouv. acq. 203, that Professor Lowe believes that it originated in the same scriptorium. It has certain Visigothic characteristics. The ms. contains numerous medical texts attributed to Hippocrates and Galen, an antiballomena, de leccionibus Heliodorus, and other miscellaneous treatises. For a description of the mss., with facsimiles of portions, see E. Lowe, *Codices Latini Antiqui* (Oxford, 1935), II, 12, 25.

[145] C. Daremberg, *op. cit.*, I, 259.

[146] See below, p. 121 ff.

[147] Isidore of Seville, *Etymologiae,* Book IV, contains chapters on the history of medicine, diseases, medical books, etc.

[148] Rabanus Maurus, *De Universo,* Book XVIII, has a chapter (5), of considerably smaller compass than the section in Isidore, which deals with medicine. (*P. L.,* CXI).

[149] *Ibid.,* XVIII, 5. " Morbi omnes ex quattuor nascuntur humoribus, id est, ex sanguine et felle, melancholia et phlegmate . . . ex sanguine autem et felle acutae passiones nascuntur, quas Graeci oxea vocant; phlegmate vero et melancholia veteres causae procedunt, quas Graeci chronia dicunt."

[150] *Ibid.,* XVIII, 5. Rabanus' comparison of the various kinds of leprosy (red, white, etc.) to types of sin, is ridiculous. Concerning mandrake, he wrote: " Mandragora propter multimoda medicaminum genera sanctorum virtutibus comparatur." *Ibid.,* XIX, 8.

[151] *Ibid.,* VI, 1, contains a treatise " De Homine et Partibus Eius " which gives a rational description of the human body. Of uncertain authorship is the *Glossae Latini-Barbaricae de Partibus Humani Corporis* (*P. L.,* CXII, 1575). Most of the entries are Latin. This is followed by a *Nomina Mensium Theodiscam.*

[152] Lupus, *Epistolae,* viii (edited by L. Levillain, *Correspondence,* Paris, 1927).

[153] *Ibid.,* lxv. " Capitis autem dolorem nepoti meo parcitas potus

forsitan detrahet, si eius appetentior fuerit deprehensus. Alioqui nostro curandus reservabitur medico, qui omnes quarum nullam non ignorat, depellere se posse confidit infirmitates."

[154] J. Mabillon, *Annales Ordinis Sancti Benedicti* (Paris, 1703 ff.), III, 437. ". . . ac medicamenta eis dari praecipit, praefatus ea simul morbo tentatus antea nihil profuisse."

[155] For instance, in three letters (ep. 216, 218, 221; *M. G. H. Ep.* IV), he refers to the fevers with which he was afflicted, as a divine castigation ("ad castigandum"; "Deus . . . castigavit me post pascha multa febrium flagellatione"; "febrium castigatio"). But, on the other hand, fevers, eye trouble ("nostros oculos nebulosa . . . caliginare fecit"), and general infirmities ("senectute et infirmitate," "ingravescente infirmi corporis flebilitate") are mentioned in a number of letters without reference to spiritual causation. See ep. 44, 55, 114, 149, 154, 170, 171, 225, 238, 249). In several cases medical or pathological similes are employed in describing spiritual decadence, heresies, etc., Ep. 237, for example, compares the slight of a friend to a wound, and carries out the simile of healing as follows: "Vulnerasti siquidem cor meum sed si tempus *medendi* adhuc fieri valeat, *sana vulnus* caritatis *calamo* . . . *pigmentarum* genera . . ." The citations given, refer to the letter numbers as given in *M. G. H. Ep.* Alcuin's letters as given in *P. L.,* C, have an entirely different numbering; in this edition the following letters contain references to diseases or medicine: ep. xxxii, xxxvi, xxxvii, lvi, lxv, lxxxiv, lxxxviii, xcvi, cvi, cxxviii, cxxix, cxxx, cxxxiv, cli, clv, clxxiii, clxxx. The constant references to ailments and medical affairs in Alcuin's works suggest that he suffered much from ill health, and that, in spite of his outwardly spiritual attitude, he was familiar with the various aspects of human medicine. The same medical-mindedness crops out occasionally in the works of Alcuin's contemporaries. Among those examples seldom mentioned in medical histories, is the letter from Paulinus, Patriarch of Aquileia to Charles the Great (ep. 17; *M. G. H. Ep.,* IV, 523), in which the tribulations of his life are described in terms such as the following: "internarum viscerum meorum vitalia . . .

toxifluo . . . vitiato pulmone . . . mei stomachi refrigerasse . . . purgato igitur iecore mentis ysopi asparso . . . cataplasmato . . ."

[156] Alcuin, *Didascalia,* de rhetorica et virtutibus (*P. L.,* CI, 947). "Medicina est scientia curationum ad temperamentum et salutem corporis inventa." Compare this with the almost identical definition given by Bishop Ermenric of Passau in a letter to Abbot Grimaldus of St. Gall, late in the ninth century (*M. G. H. Ep.,* V, 541), and with Rabanus Maurus' description in *de Universo,* XVIII, 5.

[157] Ep. 281 (*M. G. H. Ep.,* IV). "Italia infirma est patria, et escas generat noxias, idcirco cautissima consideratione videas quid, quando, vel qualiter, vel quibus utaris cibis, et maxime ebrietatis assiduitatem devita, quia ex vini calore febrium ardor ingruere solet super incautos."

[158] Ep. XXXVI (*P. L.,* C). "Sunt quaedam infirmitates quae melius dulcioribus medicantur potionibus quam amaris, et quaedam quae melius amarioribus quam dulcibus."

[159] Ep. 213 (*M. G. H. Ep.,* IV). "Solent namque medici ex multorum speciebus pigmentorum in salutem poscentis quoddam medicamenti conponere genus, nec se ipsos fateri praesumunt creatores herbarum vel aliarum specierum ex quarum compositione salus efficitur egrotantium, sed ministros esse in colligendo et in unum pigmentaria manu conficiendo corpus." In similarly approving fashion, one of Alcuin's contemporaries, Bishop Halitgarius of Cambrai, wrote of the varied activities of physicians: "Nam et corporum medici diversa medicamenta componunt ut, aliter vulnera, aliter morbum, aliter tumores, aliter putredines . . . aliter confractiones . . ." *Liber Poenitentialis* (*P. L.,* CV, 706). J. Laforêt, *Histoire d'Alcuin* (Paris, 1898), p. 132, quotes the following letter from Alcuin, but I have been unable to locate it in any of the editions. "Legimus in saecularis literaturae historiis, quosdam viros medicinalis artis peritos, dum aliquas civitates pestilentiae infectas audierunt, amore civium suorum, aliquod medicamenti genus provida sollicitudine excogitasse quo cives suos a grassantis morbi infestione praemunirent, ne ingruens periculum ex insperato partem cognatae subverterit multitudinis."

[160] Alcuin, *Carmina* XXVI (*M. G. H., Poetae*, I).

> " Accurunt medici mox Hippocratica tecta
> Hic venas fundit, herbas hic miscet in olla,
> Ille coquit pultes, alter sed pocula praefert
> Et tamen, O medici, cunctis impendite gratis
> Ut manibus vestris adsit benedictio Christi."

[161] To the Abbot of Aniane, he wrote: "*Herbas medicinales* quas direxisti, gratanti animo accepi. . . . Nam infirmus suam desiderat sanitatem, sicut et medicus . . ." Ep. 56 (*M. G.H. Ep.,* IV). In ep. 171, appears a reference to herbs: " Per campos colles herbas. . . . Hippocratis campos . . . peragrare." See also ep. 237 (*calamo, pigmentarum*).

[162] Epigrammate, 222, *De cella in eremo* (*P. L.,* CI, 1431).

> " Prate salutiferis florebunt omnia et herbis,
> Quas medici quaerit dextra salutis ope."

[163] Alcuin, *Epistolae,* 45. "Nam Basilius medicus, qui vobis in montanis Romam pergenti medicamenta tradidit, jam mortuus est." See also *Epistolae,* 77, concerning a " negotiatorem Italiae mercimonia ferentem"; and above, note 99, concerning imported herbs.

[164] *De Poenitentia,* IV, 26 (*P. L.,* CV). Non liceat in collectione herbarum, quae medicinales sunt, aliquas observationes vel incantationes attendere, nisi tantum cum symbolo divino et oratione Dominica, ut Deus et Dominus honoretur."

[165] *De Universo,* XVIII, 5. . . . "qui pigmenta et antidota satis vel assidue biberint, vexantur."

[166] Einhard, *Vita Karoli,* xxii (*M. G. S.,* II). "Et tunc quidem plura suo arbitratu quam medicorum consilio faciebat, quos pene exoses habebat, quod ei incibis assa quibus assuetus erat, dimittere, et elixis assuescere suadebant."

[167] *Ibid.,* xxiv. " In cibo et potu temperans, sed in potu temperantior, quippe ebrietatem in qualicumque homine, nedum in se ac suis plurimum abhominabatur. Cibo enim non adeo abstinere poterat, ut saepe quereretur, noxia corpori suo esse ieiunia. Convivabatur rarissime, et hoc praecipuis tantum festivitatibus, tunc tamen cum magno hominum numero. Caena cotidiana quaternis

tantum ferculis praebebatur, praeter assam, quam venatores veribus inferre solebant. . . . Vini et omnis potus adeo parcus in bibendo erat, ut super caenam raro plus quam ter biberet. Aestate post cibum meridianum pomorum aliquid sumens, ac semel bibens, depositis vestibus et calcamentis, velut noctu solitus erat, duabus aut tribus horis quiescebat. . . . *Ibid.*, xxii. Delectabatur etiam vaporibus aquarum naturaliter calentium, frequenti natatu corpus exercens, cuius adeo peritus fuit, ut nullus ei iuste valeat anteferri. Ob hoc etiam Aquisgrani regiam extruxit. . . . "

[168] See above, p. 42 ff.

[169] Einhard, *Vita Karoli,* xxii. " Per quatuor annos crebro febribus corripiebatur. Cumque ibi hyemaret, mense Januario, febre valida correptus decubuit. Qui statim, ut in febribus solebat, cibi sibi abstinentiam indixit, arbitratus hac continentia morbum posse depelli vel certe mitigari; sed accedente ad febrem lateris dolore, quem Graeci pleuresin vocant, sustentante, septimo postquam decubuit die sacra communione percepta decessit."

[170] Einhard, *Epistolae,* xiii-xiv (*M. G. H. Epistolae,* V). " Cognoscere dignetur piissima domina nostra, quod ego servus vester, postquam de Aquis exivi, tantis corporis incommodis affectus sum ut de Traiecto vix decimo die pervenire possem ad Valentianas. Ibi me tam magnus renium simul ac splenas dolor invasit ut ne unum quidem miliarium in integro die valeam equitando conficere. . . . Deus testis est, quod de infirmitate mea nullam falsitatem vobis scripsi; et non solum hoc, sed etiam quod multo graviora sunt, alia quedam incommoda, quae patior in nemetipso, de quibus nisi cum fidelissimo nullam possum habere locutionem. . . . Si me imbecillitas corporis non impediret, non has litteras mitterem, sed potius ipse venirem. . . . Inde, qui iam equitare non valui . . . navigavi. Nam et nimia ventris solutio et renium dolor sic in me alternando sibi succedunt ut nulla dies fuerit, postquam de Aquis promovi, quin hac vel illa infirmitate laborarem. Sunt pariter hec et alia que mihi ex illo morbo, in quo anno preterito iacui, contigerant, dextri videlicet femoris continuus torpor ac splenas pene intolerabilis dolor. His passionibus affectus, valde tristem ac pene omni iucunditate carentem duco vitam."

[171] Einhard, *Annales,* an. 817 (*P. L.,* CIV). ". . . imi pectoris pars sinistra contusa est, et auris dextra in parte posteriore vulnerata, femur quoque dextrum cuiusdam ligni pondere iuxta inguina conlisum. Sed instantia medicorum qui ei curam adhibebant, summa celeritate convaluit. Nam vicesima postquam id acciderat die . . . venatu sese exercebat."

[172] See above, notes 62 and 128.

[173] See above, note 122.

[174] See above, note 153.

[175] Lupus, *Epistolae,* lxviii. "Artis vestrae singularis peritia multorum ore pervulgata fratris Nithardi potissimum relatione nobis innotuit. . . . Namque et filii nostri quos et vestros optamus molestia corporis laborabant; quam aliquot adhibiti apud nos medici propulsare nequiverunt. Hos, Domino et vestrae caritati fidentes, curandos vobis offerimus. . . ."

[176] The physicians mentioned above (notes 159, 160, 166) may have been laymen. The same is possible of Wintarus, Charles the Great's physician, who is referred to as follows in *Vita Sancti Sturmi,* xxiv (*M. G. S.,* II, 377; also *P. L.,* CV): ". . . habito secum medico domini regis Karoli, cui nomen Wintarus, qui eius subveniret infirmitati. Dum vero quadam die artis suae ei nescio quam potionem infuderat, cum qua minuere debuit infirmitatem, sed ita auxit, ut validius et acrius ei lues acerba augeretur." Alcuin seems to have made reference to the same person (ep. 8, *M. G. H. Ep.,* IV) when he mentioned "Uinter medicus mihi promisit duo carrata de vino optimo et claro. . . ." Grimaldus, "bajulis et comitis sacri palatii," during Carolingian times, and author of a treatise *de dieta ciborum et nutritura ancipitrum* (Poitiers, ms. 184, f. 70-3), may not have been a physician, but he was apparently a layman.

[177] See above, p. 52; also *Histoire Littéraire de la France* (Paris, 1733 ff.), V, 608.

[178] *Gesta Episcoporum Tullensium,* xxix (*M. G. S.,* VIII). "Insuper adquisivit ab Everelmo *regali medico* in Isciaco mansos 4 et dimidium cum ecclesia. . . ."

[179] See above, p. 70; also Dill, *op. cit.*, p. 241 ff., H. Graetz, *History of the Jews* (Philadelphia, 1891 ff.), III, 35 and *passim.*; I. Munz, *Die Jüdischen Aerzte im Mittelalter* (Frankfurt, 1922), pp. 61 ff.

[180] Graetz, *op. cit.*, III, 170; Neuburger, *op. cit.*, II, part I, 276. Neuburger accepts the rather common assertion that Charles the Great's emissary (or perhaps interpreter), Isaac the Jew, who accompanied the embassy to Haroun al Raschid's court, was a physician. I have found no contemporary evidence of this fact.

[181] See the *Jewish Encyclopedia,* VIII, 415-16; Graetz, *op. cit.*, III, 35, 242, concerning the Jews in Spain and Italy; also Neuburger, *op. cit.*, II, part I, 276-7, concerning Donnolo the Italian Jew; and I Munz., *op. cit.*, p. 61 ff.

[182] Rabanus Maurus, *de Clericorum Institutione,* III, 1 (*P. L.,* CVII, 377). "Nec enim eis aliqua eorum ignorare licet . . . id est scientiam Sanctarum Scripturarum . . . [et] differentiam medicaminum, contra varietatem aegritudinum."

[183] *Capit. Missi, in Theodonis Villa,* vii (*M. G. H. Leges,* Sect. II, vol. I, 15, 121). "De medicinali arte, ut infantes hanc discere mittantur."

[184] For instance, Alcuin, in his *Didascalia: Dialogus de Rhetorica et Virtute* (*P. L.,* CI, 947), treated medicine as one of the seven divisions of *physica,* which seems to have been identical with the quadrivium; viz., it consisted of "arithmetica, astronomia, astrologia, mechanica, *medicina,* geometria, musica." About a half century later, Bishop Ermenrich of Passau wrote concerning the divisions of *physica* in identical terms (*Epistolae,* in *M. G. H., Epistolae,* V, 541). Dungal the Irishman went a step further and not only mentioned medicine as one of the liberal arts, but dedicated to it several lines of poetical description. I quote the opening lines inasmuch as they illustrate an unusual usage (for that time) of the term *physica*; viz., as synonymous with *medicina.*

> "Lucida quae cernis clarescere tecta, viator,
> Si *medicina* tibi est opus, hospes odi,
> Hic quia odoriferis circumdata tympora sertis

Ipsa salutifera munera tractat ovans.
Quam repperit primus *phisicae* tractor Apollo,
Cum quo Scolaphius, natus hic ille pater."

Dungal, *De Artibus Liberalibus,* ix (*M. G. H., Poetae,* I, 408).
Ordinarily, *physica* was used in a broader sense. See Neuburger,
op. cit., II, part I, 270; and Dubreuil-Chambardel, *op. cit.,* p.
220 ff., for general remarks concerning medicine as a part of the
liberal arts curriculum. It might also be noted that Theodulf, in
his *Carmina,* line 108 (*M. G. H., Poetae,* I, 629), refers to
physica as an *ars socia* of the liberal arts.

[185] Isidore, *op. cit.,* IV, 13. " Quaeritur a quibusdam quare
inter ceteras liberales disciplinas medicinae ars non contineatur.
Propterea quia illae singulares continent causas, ista vera omnium.
Nam et grammaticam medicus scire debet ut intellegere vel ex-
ponere possit quae legit. Similiter et rhetoricam ut veracibus
argumentis valeat definire quae tractat. Necnon et dialecticam
propter infirmitatum causas ratione adhibita perscrutandas atque
curandas. sic et arithmeticam propter numerum horarum in acces-
sionibus et periodis dierum. Nam aliter et geometriam propter
qualitates regionum et locurum situs, in quibus doceat quid quisque
observare oporteat. Porro musica incognita illi non erit nam multa
sunt quae in aegris hominibus per hanc disciplinam facta leguntur.
. . . Postremo et astronomiam notam habebit, per quam con-
templetur rationem astrorum et mutationem temporum. Nam
sicut ait quidam medicorum, cum ipsorum qualitatibus et nostra
corpora commutantur, Hinc est quod medicina secunda philosphia
dicitur. Utraque enim disciplina totum hominem sibi vindicat.
Nam sicut per illam anima ita per hanc corpus curatur."

[186] Above, pp. 52 f., 77 f.

[187] Paris B. N. 11218 and 11219 are compilations of miscellaneous medical treatises, thrown together in rather haphazard
fashion (cf. the tables of contents given below). B. N. 6880 is
the chief existing ms. of Marcellus *de medicamentis.* It is preceded by a number of medical letters and minor excerpts; e. g.,
f. 2 de mensuris et ponderibus medicinalibus ex Greco translatis

iuxta Hyppocratis; f. 4 epistolae diversorum de qualitate et observatione medicinae. . . . Largius designatianus. . . . Antiocho regi Hippocrates . . . ep. alia eiusdem Hippocrates ex Greco translata ad Maecenatem . . . ep. Plinii Secundi ad amicos de medicina . . . ep. Cornelius Celsus G. Jul. Calisto . . . ep. Cornelius Celsus Pullio natali . . . ; f. 28-9, 33, 35, and 42 contain stray remedies, and f. 150 has verses quod natum Phoebus docuit. . . . Paris B. N. ms. 12995, f. 1-197 is an excellent version of Dioscorides de virtutibus herbarum arranged in the usual five books. Angers ms. 457 (442) contains Alexander of Tralles de morbis in three books (f. 1-138) and his de pulsibus et urinis (f. 140-2). Inasmuch as mss. 11218 and 11219 contain a great many treatises which are not adequately listed in the catalogues, I am giving the titles (and in some cases brief incipits) of all treatises of both mss. The following is the list of contents of B. N. ms. 11218: f. 1 (computus table); f. 2 (vita of a saint); f. 6 epitome periodeotecon; f. 8 (passionarius) de peripleomonia . . . ; f. 11 (antidotary) antidotum Teodorico . . . electuario . . . ; f. 12 (passionarius) de cause epatice . . . ; f. 16 epistula Accii Justi [cf. with B. N. 203, f. 22; and St. Gall, 751, p. 356]; f. 21 ep. de quattuor partes corpus. Eppocratis ad Antioco rege . . . [cf. B. N. 11219, f. 41]; f. 23 (The seven ages of man) Singulas etatis . . . ; f. 24 (passionarius) desenteria colera . . . ; f. 26 ep. Ypograti de indicium medicine artis. . . . Prima medicinalis racio est . . . ; f. 28 de urinis; f. 30 ep. Vindiciano ad Pentadioni nepotem de quattuor humoribus . . . [cf. B. N. 11219, f. 18 and 103]; f. 32 (passionarius) ad cardis doloris . . . ; f. 33 ep. conflictus duorum filosoporum . . . in quo humores . . . ; f. 34 ep. fleobotomie. quid est fleobotomia . . . [cf. Montpellier 185, f. 98]; f. 37 explicit ep. Eliodori digitorum manus operacio; f. 37 ep. Gallieni de febrientibus . . . ; f. 39 (hermeneumata) Hermeguma i. e., interpretatio pimentorum vel herbarum; f. 42 (herbal) nomine erbe botracion . . . ; f. 42 racio ponderum; f. 42. dogmida Epogratis et Galieni et Surani. Ubi cogitaverunt de vita et corpus . . . ; f. 43 (antidotary); f. 49 (passionarius) de epelenticus . . .

de capite . . . ; f. 56 hic est virtus de duodecim mensibus; f. 57 antidotum tussentibus . . .; f. 57 liber confeccionarius. (antidotary in two books) ; f. 100 de signa mortalia; f. 101 de disposicione de lunas; f. 101 signa si eger(?) moriturus est aut vitalis; f. 102 (antidotary) pucione ad ebrugine . . .; f. 111 (passionarius) de apoplexia secta [secundum?] Gallieni . . . explicit oxiarum; f. 113 (antidotary) confectio ad paralisim . . .; f. 115 de etate hominis [cf. Chartres 80 (ninth-tenth century), f. 45-47]; f. 115-826 (antidotary) antidotum que usus est Theodosius. . . . Of somewhat similar content is B. N. 11219: f. 1 (Hippocrates) Aforismi; f. 12 liber epistol . . . ep. quod per omnes curas adhibenda sint medicamenta . . . ep. Primitus legenda de disciplina artis medicinae . . . ep. Arsenii ad Nepotianum . . . ep. de ratione organi . . . ep. Ypogratis de observatione temporum . . . prologus Gallieni de sanguine et flegma . . . de tempore anni . . . ep Ypogratis de quatuor humoribus . . . ep. Ypocratis ad Mecenatem. Provocas me . . . ; f. 20 Epistola Ysagogus . . . tractatus Ysagogus. . . . In acutibus passionibus . . . ; f. 24 de passionibus unde eveniunt. Frenetica . . . ; f. 26 liber interrogationis Yppogratis medici. Quid est medicina . . . ; f. 29 de balneis . . . ; f. 32 insomnis . . . ; f. 32 ep. flevotomiae. Quid est flebotomia . . . f 33 ep flevotomis; f. 34 ep. flevotomia. Cirurgia dicitur . . . ; f. 35 ep. de incisione flevotomi quam composuit Yppocratis . . . ; f. 36 ferramentorum nomina. Necesse est universorum ferramentorum nomina diceret . . . ; f. 36 cirurgia Eliodori. Cirurgie operatio . . . ; f. 38 de signa mortifera iuxta Yppogratis sanientiam; f. 38 (passionarius) Nunc faciem dicendum in hoc libro superum de aliis dicturus causis in alio quippiam i. e., de fleomonium . . .; f. 39 de interrogatione medicinali. Quare badamus . . . ; f. 39 Quatuor sunt venti . . . f. 41 ep. Ypocratis ad Antiocum et Antonium de quatuor membrorum . . . ; (passionarius) Tereoperica hoc est liber medicinalis scriptus specialiter secundum philosoforum auctorei inquisitiones . . . ; (103 chapters); f. 103 ep. Ipocratis et Galieni contemplantis quatuor est humores . . . ; f. 104 liber medicinalis de omni corpore hominis Terapeutica. Hoc est collectum ex libris multis philosophorum specialiter a capite . . . (110 chapters with interpolations; e. g., antidotary fragment on f. 141, brevem ad demonium expellendum on f. 143; from f. 145 on, ch. 88 ff. deal with confectiones, unguentes, etc.); f. 169 (monthly observationes) mens mars bibat dulce . . . ; f. 169 pronostica de mortibus (cf. Chartres ms. 62 f. 38); f. 169 (continuation of passionarius) de frenesim . . . de emorroide . . . ; f. 171 Hermeneumata id est interpretatio pigmentorum . . . (cf. Paris B. N. 11218, f. 39); (Egyptian Days); f. 179 Hermeneumata de decim speciebus medicamentibus; f. 191 de potu . . . aqua . . . vinum . . . olerum . . . ; f. 192 de signis ponderum secundum Grecos . . . ; f. 192 de propriis nominibus arborum; . . . de herbis aromaticis . . . de odoratis holeribus . . . ; f. 207 de herbis Galieni Apollonii et Ciceronis; f. 210 Actio Justi medici de muliebria . . . ; f. 212 ep. Ypocratis ad Micanetem. LI Provocas me de studio. . . . LII incipit prologus. . . . LIII incipit liber primus de offocatio contingat de matrices subito . . . (and so on ch. LIIII to LXXXVI; evidently a portion of a passionarius); f. 221-33 (antidotary) pulvera probatissima . . . antebalumina Galieni.

[188] See above, note 143.

[189] In Paris at the B. N. are the following: ms. 12958, f. 67-73 a fragment of Galen's Prosglaucon, book I; ms. 9347, f. 49-57 a fragment (from Rheims) of Quintus Serenus Sammonicus' liber medicinalis; ms. nouv. acq., 1613, f. 12 a fragment of Quintus Serenus Sammonicus, f. 4 and 21 treatises on weights and measures; ms. nouv. acq., 1616, f. 10-12 a treatise on Egyptian Days, and f. 14 miscellaneous remedies; ms. 5240 contains one folio (f. 116) of remedies de febribus; ms. 13013, f. 1 and 29 adjuratio versus febres; ms. 13403, f. 113-18 an almost illegible de medicina; and ms 10251, f. 70-102 liber medicinalis. From the departmental libraries comes only one ms., Laon 420; it contains letters from Hippocrates (?) ad Mecenatem, and Antiocho regi.

[190] With only a few exceptions the treatises and writers mentioned in this paragraph are to be found in the five mss. of which

analyses are given above in note 187. Most of them are from mss. B. N. 11218 and 11219. The *Liber Medicinalis* of Quintus Serenus Sammonicus (in verse) is from B. N. 9347, f. 49-57 and B. N. nouv. acq., 1613, f. 12. Other minor or fragmentary works are found in the mss. analysed in note 189.

[191] Paris B. N. nouv. acq. 203, f. 2. For an analysis of this ms. see above, note 144. Note 187 has a description of ms. B. N. 11218; see especially folio 16.

[192] See above, p. 74 ff.

[193] See above, note 86.

[194] See above, note 98, concerning the St. Gall infirmary.

[195] In 816 the Council of Aix-la-Chapelle (ch. 142), in its regulations (de infirmorum ac senum cura fratrum) concerning cathedral canons, decreed that there should be a " mansio infirmorum et senum intra claustra canonicorum" in each center. *M. G. H. Leges,* Sectio III, II, 417. A few years later (845), another French council (Meldense, ch. 53) decreed as follows: " ut canonici in *civitate vel monasteriis,* sicut constitutum est, in dormitorio dormiant, in refectario comedant, et in *domo infirmorum* necessaria subleventur." Mansi, *Concilia* . . . XIV, 831. From the later middle ages (Liber Ord. S. Victor Paris., ch. 40), we have the following illustration of the complicated infirmary service that had developed. In the infirmaria there were three types of patients; namely, " qui lecto prorsus decubant . . . qui de infirmitate convalescunt . . . qui huiusmodi infirmitatem non habent ut tamen in infirmaria assidue comedunt . . . ut senes, caeci. . . ." Du Cange, *Glossarium,* III, 825.

[196] The Hôtel Dieu at Paris is said to have been restored by Charles the Great, and there were throughout Northern France Hospitalia Scotorum, the restoration and protection of which was decreed in 845 at the Council of Meaux (ch. 40), Mansi, *Concilia,* XIV, 827. See also the article on hospitals in the Catholic Encyclopedia, and below, note 197, for the numerous decrees of Carolingian times concerning the general restoration, and protection of already existing institutions.

[197] There are passages concerning tithes, "elymosyna," "hospitalitate," "hospitio," "hospitale," "xenodochia," etc., that were to be set apart for the care of the "pauperes," "peregrini," etc., in the following capitularies: capitularies of the years 789 (ch. 9), 801 (ch. 7), 802 (ch. 27, 29), 803 (ch. 3), in *M. G. S.* III, 68, 87, 94, 110); and also for the years 809 (ch. 35), and 819 (ch. 5), in *Rec. Hist. Fr.*, V, 68; VI, 429. Passages of similar import are to be found in the following records of church councils: Leptines (743), Aix-la-Chapelle (816), and Aix-la-Chapelle (836). See Sudhoff, ". . . Geschichte d. Krankenhauswesens . . .", *loc. cit.*, p. 195; also *M. G. H. Leges*, sectio II, I, 28; sectio III, II, part I, 7, and part II, 416, 455. In like manner, other types of sources (e. g., letters, charters, etc.,) contain references to hospices and charity service. There are numerous instances of "hospitalia nobilium" and "hospitalia pauperum"; see *Rec. Hist. Fr.*, IX, 350; J. Thillier et E. Jarry, *Cartulaire de Ste.-Croix d'Orléans* (Paris, 1906), p. 82; *Miracula S. Benedicti*, ch. 23; C. Cuissard, *Théodulfe Evêque d'Orléans* (Orleans, 1892), p. 262; and Du Cange, *Glossarium*, III, 702-3. So far as letters are concerned, one example will suffice. Pope Hadrian I (ep. 30), wrote to Charles the Great urging the protection and preservation of a monastery "cum *hospitalibus* qui per colles Alpium siti sunt *pro peregrinorum* susception." (*Rec. Hist. Fr.*, V, 585). The Carolingian sources concerning hospices contain many references to the recognized Christian duty of hospitality, which we believe was the chief factor in the establishment of such institutions. The clerical function of providing "hospitalitas" for "pauperis" and "peregrini" is mentioned in the following: Council of Tours (813), ch. 6; Council of Arles (813), ch. 17; Council of Rheims (813), ch. 17; and Council of Aix-la-Chapelle (836), I, ch. 3. See *M. G. H. Leges*, sectio III, II, part I; and Mansi, *Concilia*, XIV, 671 ff.; also Du Cange, *Glossarium*, III, 702 ff., for Latin passages concerning hospices, hospitality, etc.; and below, note 202, concerning the varied charitable services performed at Theodulph's Orleans hospice.

[198] E. Withington, *Medical History from the Earliest Times* (London, 1894), p. 182.

[199] M. Neuburger, *op. cit.*, II, part I, 327.

[200] See above note 141 concerning Merovingian councils, and note 197, concerning the councils at Leptines (743), and Aix-la-Chapelle (816 and 836). The action taken at these councils seems to have been a part of the effort to restore monastic life to the former Benedictine regime. At Leptines, for instance, it was decreed that " Abbates et monachi receperunt Sancti Patris Benedicti [regulam] ad restaurandam norman regularis vitae." *M. G. H. Leges,* sectio II, I, 28.

[201] The men of the Carolingian age defined hospices as " xenodochia in quibus sit quotidiana *pauperum* et *peregrinorum* susceptio," or as " domus ubi *peregrini* vel *miseri* recipiuntur in hospitium." (Sudhoff, ". . . Geschichte d. Krankenhauswesens . . .", *loc. cit.*, p. 195; Du Cange, *Glossarium,* III, 702). It is unfortunate from the standpoint of accuracy that the medieval term " hospitalia " is so often translated as " hospital." This literal transcription results in serious misrepresentation. Note, for instance, the chapter on hospitals in J. Walsh, *Medieval Medicine*; the references in O. Dalton, *The History of the Franks by Gregory of Tours,* I, 347; the articles on hospitals in the *Catholic Encyclopedia,* and in F. Cabrol et H. Leclercq, *Dictionnaire d'Archéologie Chrétienne et de Liturgie* (Paris, 1923). In these works, and in many others, the great majority of the examples cited as " hospitals " are in actual fact hospices; and there is no clear indication of the fact that hospices were fundamentally non-medical. K. Sudhoff, " Geschichte d. Krankenhauswesens . . .", *loc. cit.*, and M. Neuburger, *op. cit.*, II, part I, 327, in gratifying contrast, make clear the distinction between " guest houses " and " sick houses." Neither, however, has any detailed information concerning French hospices.

[202] Theodulf, *Carmina,* lix (*M. G. H., Poetae,* I, 554).

> " Et patet ista domus mediocri exacta paratu,
> Utcumque humanis usibus apta tamen . . .
> Esuriens epulas, sitiens potum, hospes honorem;
> Nudus operimentum hic reperire queat.
> Fessus opem, *languens medicamen,* gaudia maestus

Hinc ferat, et cunctis consulat ista domus.
Det pater altithronus donum hoc habitantibus istic,
Civibus ut pateat, *et peregrini,* tibi,
Ut fratrum atque dei regnet dilectio semper,
Virtutesque omnes hac duce conveniant . . ."

[203] H. Taylor, *The Medieval Mind* (New York, 1911), I, 211.

[204] E. Littré, *op. cit.,* p. 263.

CHAPTER III

[205] See the excellent summary of this problem by G. Burr, " The Year 1000 and the Antecedents of the Crusades," *Am. Hist. Rev.,* VI (1901), 429 ff. J. Roy, *L'an Mille* . . . (Paris, 1885) has a good bibliography of works on the subject.

[206] E. Joranson, *The Danegeld in France,* gives a constructive interpretation of this era.

[207] H. Waddell, *The Wandering Scholars* (New York, 1928), p. 64; quoting the nineteenth century historian Trench and the eleventh century chronicler Rodulfus Glaber.

[208] A. Clerval, *Les Ecoles de Chartres au Moyen Age* (Paris, 1895), p. 1 ff.

[209] *Ibid.,* p. 1-2; citing Julius Caesar, *de Bello Gallico,* VI, 13-14; Lucan, *Pharsalia,* I, 440; and Pliny, *Historia Naturalis,* XVI, 44.

[210] B. Guérard, *Cartolaire de l'abbaye de Saint-Père de Chartres* (Paris, 1840), I, p. lxix.

[211] See C. Daremberg and M. Bussemaker, *Oeuvres d'Oribase* (Paris, 1851 ff.), VI, p. xv ff., for A. Molinier's description of the Latin translations of Oribasius. Certain points in this description are open to criticism; for instance, the assertion that mss. B. N. 10233 and 9332 " ont été très certainement exécutés en *Italie."* Several eminent paleographers have corroborated my opinion that both mss. are of French origin. For a recent and dependable analysis of the mss. see H. Moerland, *Die Lateinischen Oribasius Über-setzungen* (Oslo, 1932), pp. 11 ff. Moerland dates ms. 10233 fifth-sixth century; Molinier dates it sixth-seventh; Diels (*op. cit.,* II, 72) and Delisle (Cabinet, II, 11), seventh; E. Chatelain, *Uncialis*

Scriptura Latinorum (Paris, 1901), p. 99, dates it eighth century. See also below, note 219, for the curiously different datings that have been given to the Paris and Berne portions of the ms.

[212] For the minor treatises in this ms. see above, note 144; they follow the nine *libri Oribasii* (f. 1-263) and the *Rufus de Podagra* (f. 263-71). The ms. is not complete; quaternions xviii-xxiii inclusive, (comprising the last part of Oribasius book V, and all of book VI) are missing. This material, which should be between f. 134 and f. 135, is to be found in part in a Berne ms. of fragments (see below note 219); only the chapters from book V are contained in this fragment. So far as is known, book VI is not extant. Similar to the Oribasius text of B. N. 10233, is that in a seventh-eighth century ms., B. N. nouv. acq. 1619. This ms., originally from Troyes, contains eight books of Oribasius (f. 1-206). See Moerland, *op. cit.,* p. 12, for an analysis. The material which comprises book IV differs from that in B. N. 10233; the subject matter of the last three books is the same in both mss., but they are numbered VI, VII, VIII in ms. 1619, and VII, VIII, VIIII in ms. 10233. Apparently ms. 10233 had an additional book, the missing book VI. Ms. 1619 has several minor treatises; viz., a glose de mensuras and an ermenguma (i. e., hermeneumata) (f. 178); and at the end of the ms. (f. 206-7) are remedies ad morbo regio, pocio aposmtcis, etc.

[213] Ms. 9332 contains the following: eight books of Oribasius (of which the first three differ considerably from ms. 10233, but are identical to ms. 1619; and of which the last is numbered book VIII); f. 138-321 contain Alexander of Tralles and Dioscorides, but the end of the former and the beginning of the latter are missing. The *Therapeutica* of Alexander, in three books, begins with a table of chapters and a full page illumination (see plate III); books I and II are complete, but book III has only the table of chapters and 66 chapters of the text. Between f. 242 and f. 243 six folios are missing. This is evident from the fact that the original foliation of the ms. (in Roman numerals) omits folios mcxlviiii-mcliv inclusive. The missing folios contained not only the last two chapters of Alexander's third book, but also the table of contents

and chapters i-xxxii of book I of the *Materia Medica* of Dioscorides. Dioscorides books II-V are complete (they and the ms. end with f. 321). The following minor treatises are inserted in the ms.: f. 251 epistula uulter. Provinciae Babiloniae Alexandriae regis Romae salutem. Nescit humanus genus quantam virtutem habit uultor . . .; f. 233 ad demonio expellendo . . .; f. 321 (at the end of Dioscorides book V), ad morbo regio, which is followed by three lines in a later hand (tenth century?), Ocrm Concordia . . .

[214] L. Delisle, *Cabinet des Manuscrits de la Bibliothèque Nationale* . . . (Paris, 1868 ff.), II, 11.

[215] *Ibid.*, II, 11.

[216] On folio 2 of the ms. itself is a notation, in a modern hand, which reads " septimum "; but this has been crossed out and above it, in another hand, is the number " VIII." Puhlman, *op. cit.*, p. 399, and Delisle, *op. cit.*, II, 11 (also in the Inventaire of mss. of the B. N.), date it ninth century; Moerland, *op. cit.*, p. 11, suggests eighth-ninth century. For similar variations in dating mss., see below, note 219 concerning B. N. 10233 and Berne F. 219.

[217] See Clerval, *op. cit.*, pp. 13, 17, 23, 27. On p. 13, for instance, he writes of two religious mss. and one medical ms. (B. N. 10233) from eighth century Chartres, and concludes that " the studies of the eighth century were reduced to the Gospels, the Fathers, and medicine . . ." In like fashion W. B. Aspinwall, *Les Ecoles Episcopales et Monastiques de l'Ancienne Province Ecclésiastique de Sens du VIe au XIIe Siècle* (Paris, 1904), p. 20. In none of the monographs or general works on the subject have I found any expression of doubt as to these mss. being ample evidence of medical studies in Chartres.

[218] Professor Beeson, in response to my question concerning B. N. 9332, writes, " I should never have thought of Chartres as the schriftheimat of the ms."; and " I am inclined to assign the ms. to Fleury." Professor Lowe, while declining to locate the ms. with absolute certainty, writes; " I see nothing in the ms. that takes me to Chartres," and believes that " there may be something in the Fleury connection." So far as ms. B. N. 10233 is concerned, Pro-

fessor F. M. Carey, who has specialized on Fleury mss., writes me that " to the best of our knowledge, the ms. came from Fleury or the vicinity of Orleans."

[219] B. N. 10233, f. 120-34 contains the table of contents of Oribasius Book V, and chapter i-xxxiii of the text; Berne F. 219, no. 3, f. 15-18 contains the remainder of the text of book V (viz., chapter xxxiv-xlii). The next 16 folios of the original ms. are lost; they comprised book VI and the first part of the table of contents of book VII (chapter i-xxix). The Berne ms., f. 1-14, contains the remainder of the table of contents of book VII, and part of the text. The rest is in ms. 10233, f. 135 ff. It is possible to check the number of lost folios from the numbered quaternions in the extant sections and from the early foliation (in Roman numerals) which was made before the ms. was broken up. For instance, ms. 10233, f. 1-134, comprises Roman folios x-cxliii, i. e., quaternions I-XVII (quaternion III has 6 rather than 8 folios). The Berne ms. f. 15-18 comprises Roman folios cxliv-cxlvii, i. e., the first half of quaternion XVIII. Then comes the missing link. Berne, f. 1-14, carries on with Roman folios clxiv-clxxvii, comprising quaternions XXII-XXIII (XXIII has only 6 folios). Ms. 10233, f. 135 ff. contains Roman folios clxxviii ff., comprising quaternions XXIIII ff. The dating of these mss. is of some interest. Puhlmann, *op. cit.*, p. 399, evidently unaware of the fact that they were parts of the same ms., dates B. N. 10233 sixth-seventh century, and Berne F 219 seventh-eighth. H. Hagen, *De Oribasii Versione Latina Bernensi* (Berne, 1875), p. iii-iv, dates B. N. 10233 seventh century, and Berne F 219 sixth century. The supposition that Fleury was the place of origin of the entire ms., rests on the fact that fragments no. 1 and 2 of Berne F 219 came from the library of Pierre Daniels who had many Fleury mss.; fragment no. 3, inasmuch as it was bound with them, doubtless came from the same source, through the hands of the book collector Bongars. For the dispersion of the Fleury mss., the part played by Daniels and Bongars in collecting them, and the manner in which many of them finally turned up at Berne, see C. Cuissard, *Inventaire des manuscrits de la Bibliothèque d'Orléans*

Fonds de Fleury (Orleans, 1885), p. xxii ff. So far as the Berne fragment of Oribasius is concerned, the Daniels-Bongars theory seems probable. But the problem still remains; how can one account for the major portion of the ms. being at Chartres. At the time of the Huguenot ravages did some cleric carry it there for safety, leaving behind some 30 or more folios, which were salvaged by Daniels? At present there seems to be no definite solution to the problem.

²²⁰ Chartres ms. 40 is a Fleury ms., as is evident from the library marks. Chartres ms. 75, which contains some medical fragments and also works by Bede and Abbo of Fleury, impresses me as another possible Fleury ms.

²²¹ In both mss. are found marginal *notae* and corrections in the same hand, apparently of the tenth century; e. g., 10233 f. 65 and 9332 f. 30.

²²² Information concerning the early schools of Chartres can be found in the following: Clerval, *op. cit.*, p. 1-28; Aspinwall, *op. cit.*, p. 18-21; L. Maître, *Les Ecoles Episcopales et Monastiques . . . 768-1180* (Paris, 1924) ; and F. Cabrol et H. Leclercq, *Dictionnaire d'Archéologie Chrétienne et de Liturgie* (Paris, 1923), see " Chartres." In the ninth century, according to Paul, a monk of Chartres, the city " populosa admodum atque opulentissima inter Neustriae urbes, murorum magnitudine, edificorum pulchritudine, vel *artium liberalium studiis* habebatur famosissima." B. Guérard, *Cartulaire de Saint-Père*, I, 5.

²²³ The *medical* history of Fleury during the period in which it was the leader of North French schools (the ninth and tenth century), is almost a total blank. Theodulf, one of the leading lights of the court circle of Charles the Great, and in later life Abbot of Fleury, manifested in his writing some familiarity with medicine and the care of the sick (see above notes 184, 202). But, aside from infirmary service, neither he nor his monastery offer convincing evidence of a well developed medical science. Most of the statements concerning him in C. Cuissard, *Théodulfe Evêque d'Orléans* (Orleans, 1892), tend to hero worship. Similarly, the same authors' words concerning medical science at Fleury are exaggera-

tions; notably those in *L'Ecole de Fleury sur Loire à la fin du Xe Siècle* (Orleans, 1875), p. 11, 20; *L'Ecole Episcopale d'Orléans et l'Ecole Monastique de Fleury sur Loire au XIIe et au XIIIe Siècle* (Orleans, 1880, ms. 1637), p. 91-2; and in *Inventaire des Manuscrits de la Bibliothèque d'Orléans Fonds de Fleury* (Orleans, 1885), p. xii, xiv. However unreliable Cuissard's generalizations concerning medicine may be, he indicates in the last mentioned work the field in which evidence is to be found concerning medicine at Fleury; viz., in the manuscripts. L. Delisle, in *Notices et Extraits* (Paris, 1884), XXXI, part I, 357 ff., suggested the difficulties of the task, inasmuch as the manuscripts were dispersed and are "scattered about, at Orleans, Paris, Berne, Rome, and Ashburnham Place." Furthermore, since very few Fleury manuscripts have the library mark, the identification must await the intensive study of the character of Fleury manuscripts by paleographical specialists. Professor F. M. Carey of the University of California (Los Angeles) is at present working on the problem and it is to be hoped that he will publish at least a tentative list of Fleury manuscripts, in the near future. Meanwhile, it may be worth while to suggest that a place as advanced in the liberal arts as Fleury must have had medical manuscripts. If our conjectures as to B. N. mss. 10233 and 9332 are correct, we may assume that Fleury was an important center for the dissemination of Graeco-Latin medical works; comparable to Ravenna in Italy.

[224] Richer, *Historia*, III, 43 ff. (*M. G. S.*, III, 560 ff.; there is also a new edition of the Latin text with French translation, by R. LaTouche, of which only the first of the two volumes has appeared, Paris, 1930).

[225] Ep. cli (*P. L.*, CXXXIX; but I cite from the better edition by J. Havet, *Lettres de Gerbert* (Paris, 1889)). "Specialia tamen fratris morbo calculi laborantis plenius exequerer, si inventa a prioribus intueri liceret, Nunc particula antidoti philoanthropos ac eius scriptura contentus, tuo vitio imputa si quod paratum est ad salutem, non servando dietam (or dictam), verteris in perniciem, Nec me auctore quae medicorum sunt tractare velis, praesertim cum scientiam eorum tantum affectaverim, officium semper fugerim."

In this quotation, as in the others from Gerbert, I have endeavored to give a logical, rather than a strict, translation. For instance, in some mss. the reading is dictam rather than dietam. But dictam (i. e., " words," i. e., " instructions ") makes no sense in this context; dietam (i. e., diet) does, and I therefore take that reading.

[226] Ep. cxiv. " Molestia vestra dejecti, revelatione relevati sumus. Addidimus etiam et addemus supplicationes quas poterimus, et si quid ars medicinae labori nostro suggeret quam proxime dirigemus."

[227] Ep. clxix. " Itaque cum tibi desit artifex medendi, nobis remediorum materia, supersedimus describere ea quae medicorum peritissimi utilia judicaverint viciato jecori. Quem morbum tu corrupte, postuma, nostri apostema, Celsus Cornelius, a Grecis ΥΠΑΤΙΚΟΝ, dicit appellari."

[228] Ep. ix. " Si bene valetis gaudemus. Indigentiam vestram nostram putamus. quam patimur, ut relevetis rogamus. De morbis ac remediis oculorum Demosthenes philosophus librum edidit, qui inscribitur Ophthalmicus; eius principium si habetis, habeamus . . ." A tenth-century Bobbio catalogue lists librum I Demosthenis (Becker, op. cit., p. 69).

[229] Ep. cxxx.

[230] Ep. l; ep. clxii; in ep. lxvii there is a suggestion of technical bedside manner; viz., " Erit ergo docti viri, more boni medici mellita praeferre, ne primo gustu amaris ingestis antidotis, salutem suam formidabundus incipiat expavescere."

[231] Ep. ccviii. " Incredibili pene et nimium scelerata relatione tanto dolore affectus sum, ut lumen oculorum prope plorando amiserim. . . . Senectus mea mihi diem minatur ultimum. Latera pleurisis occupat, tinniunt aures, distillant oculi, totumque corpus continuis de pungitur stimulis. Totus his annus me in lecto a doloribus decumbentem vidit, et nunc vix resurgentem recidivi dolores alternis praecipitant diebus."

[232] Like the library of Fleury, those of medieval Rheims were badly devastated, and comparatively few mss. are extant. See H. Jadart, Les Anciennes Bibliothèques de Reims . . . (Rheims, 1891). Professor F. M. Carey, who has for years carried on researches in this field, directed me to the Rheims mss. which are now at Cambrai,

but among the very small number of Rheims mss. in that place, none are concerned with medicine during the early period. The following Rheims mss. contain only minor works, fragments, and a strikingly large proportion of exorcisms and other such semi-medical materials: Paris B. N. 8780 (a tenth century ms. with several marks "lib. sci. Remigii") is a handbook of Tironian notes (see plate VII); among the entries are many medical terms (see, f. 27 for materia medica, f. 39 for diseases, and f. 43 for "hipocratis"). At Rheims are the following semi-medical fragments; all are from the ninth, tenth, eleventh centuries. Ms. 73, f. 91, an exorcism for the eyes; ms. 382, f. 78, an exorcism for trouble with teeth; ms. 1413, f. 31, exorcisms for teeth and headache; ms. 438, f. 29 epistola Ypocratis de diebus aegyptiacus, f. 30 miscellaneous medical material in later hand; ms. 443, on binding sheet, days of the moon; ms. 1395, f. 183 three lines, viz. "aiunt medici scripsere naturis, quod si quis florem solicis vel populi mixtum atque biberit"; ms. 1390 (twelfth or thirteenth century?) verses on medicine. For B. N. ms. 9347, see plate VIII.

[233] Richer, *Historia,* IV, 50. "Ante horum captionem, diebus ferme 14, cum aviditate discendi logicam Yppocratis Choi, de studiis liberalibus saepe et multum cogitarem quadam die equitem Carnotinum in urbe Remorum positus offendi. Qui a me interrogatus quis et cuius esset, cur et unde venisset, Heribrandi clerici Carnotensis legatum esse, et Richero sancti Remigii monacho se velle loqui respondit. Ego mox amici nomen et legationis causam advertens, me quem querebat indicavi, datoque osculo semotim secessimus. Ille mox epistolam protulit, hortatoriam ad aphorismorum lectionem. Unde et ego admodum laetatus, assumpto quodam puero cum Carnotino equite, iter Carnotum arripere disposui. . . . Quo reducto et omni sollicitudine amota, in aphorismis Yppocratis vigilanter studui apud domnum Herbrandum magnae liberalitatis atque scientiae virum. In quibus cum tantum prognostica morborum accepissem, et simplex egritudinum cognitio cupienti non sufficeret, petii etiam ab eo lectionem eius libri qui inscribitur de concordia Yppocratis Galieni et Surani. Quod et

obtinui; cum eum in arte peritissimum, dinamidia farmaceutica, butanica, atque cirurgia non laterent."

[234] The three medical schools, or *sectae* as they were called, are mentioned in Isidore of Seville, *Etymologiae* (IV, 4) and other works on medicine. See my " Tenth Century Medicine . . .", *Bull. Inst. Hist. Medicine*, II (1934), 347 ff., note 30.

[235] Note that Richer refers to the book as *" eius* libri " (above, note 233). See my "Tenth Century Medicine . . ." *loc. cit.*, especially note 17.

[236] The " Oxea et Chronia " is a handbook of diseases, arranged from head to foot; viz., beginning with *de cefalea,* it deals with head diseases such as *de dentium vitia, de aurium vitia, de cataron,* etc., then chest and stomach ailments (e. g., *de tussicula, de stomachi causas, de colicis*) ; and so on to the lower extremities; *epaticis, spleneticis, ydropicis, diabetis, elefantiosis,* etc., ending with *de podagricis.* As an example of the subject matter of the individual chapters we may take that *de podagricis.* It begins with a description of the disease; viz., "Ad pedum dolorem nomen accepit podagra; quo modo astretis ab asticulis dolorem nomen sumpsit . . . Podagricorum generas ii; calida et frigida quia sic dinoscimus. Calida podagra est. . . . Contra calidam podagram, frigidis adiutoriis adhibemus; contra frigida, calidis . . . " (continuing with detailed remedies for podagra of the fingers, feet, etc.; these include amputation, blood-letting, purging, unguents, emplastra, abstinence from wine and certain foods, and the use of certain medicines).

[237] See my " Tenth Century Medicine . . . ," *loc. cit.*, p. 361 ff. for Richer's medical passages, with English translation and critical notes.

[238] The text of these notes appears in the version given in *M. G. S.*, III, and *P. L.*, CXXXVIII. " Libellum quem hoc anno praestitistis de medicina et de speciebus metallorum quando in armario simul fuimus, mihi transmitte."

[239] For comments on this point see my " Tenth Century Medicine . . .", *loc. cit.*, notes 7, 8, and 65.

[240] *Ibid.*, p. 361 ff.

[241] *Ibid.*, note 59 contains the Latin text (from *Historia,* III, 109)

and critical notes. " Nam cum vernalis elementia eodem anno rebus bruma afflictus, pro rerum natura immutato aere, Lauduni aegrotate coepit. Unde vexatus ea passione, quae colica a phisicis dicitur, in lectum decidit. Cui dolor intolerabilis in parte dextra super verenda erat; ab umbilico quoque usque ad splenem, et inde usque ad sinistrum, et sic ad anum, infestis doloribus pulsabatur. Ilium quoque ac renium iniuria nonulla erat; thenasmus assiduus; egestio sanguinae; vox aliquoties intercludebatur. Interdum frigore febrium rigebat. Rugitus intestinorum. Fastidium iuge. Ructus conationes sine effectu, ventris extensio, stomachi ardor, non deerant. . . ."

[242] Ibid., note 17.

[243] Ibid., p. 374 f. for the medical vocabulary, and note 19 for detailed references etc., concerning the location of the various terms.

[244] Richer's flare for the classical in his historical writing, is treated by R. LaTouche, " Un Imitateur de Salluste au Xe Siècle," Annales de l'Université de Grenoble (1929), VI, no. 3.

[245] See my " Tenth Century Medicine . . .", loc. cit., p. 354.

[246] Ibid., p. 374-5.

[247] Ibid., especially notes 39, 49, 56, 59, and 62.

[248] Dubreuil-Chambardel, op. cit., p. 223.

[249] De Universo, VI, 1; XIX, 8. See also above note 184.

[250] See my " Tenth Century Medicine . . .", loc. cit., p. 374-5.

[251] Reutter, " De la Médecine et de la Pharmacie en France au XIe et XIIe Siècles," Schweizerische Apotheker Zeitung, LIII (1915), p. 277 ff.

[252] P. Rambaud, La Pharmacie en Poitou (Paris, 1907).

[253] See above, note 233.

[254] This quotation is from the Chartres necrologie; viz., " obiit Herbrandus levita et canonicus B. Marie." See Clerval, op. cit., p. 25; R. Merlet et Clerval, Un Ms. Chartrain du XIe Siècle (Chartres, 1893), p. 167.

[255] Paris B. N. 9221, a copy on paper of a 987 charter (at end of ms.). See also P. Varin, Archives Administratives de la Ville de Reims (Paris, 1839, in Documents Inédits), I, 69, for a reference to a young oblate named Herbrannus who was dedicated to St.

Remi early in the tenth century. He could hardly have been living at the end of the century.

[256] Clerval, *op. cit.*, pp. 30, 129 f.; and Dubreuil-Chambardel, *op. cit.*, p. 9, take it for granted that Fulbert taught medicine to the young clerics who attended the cathedral school at Chartres. This is a purely gratuitous assumption. Like Gerbert, Fulbert knew medicine, but it is my impression that neither of them gave formal instruction in it. If they had, I feel that it would have been mentioned by some of their friends or students, or would have been referred to in some way in their correspondence.

[257] *Hymnus seu Prosa de Sancto Pantaleone* (*P. L.,* CXLI, 339). "... Duas esse medicinas Christianis novimus, unam quidem de terrenis, de supernis alteram; quarum ut diversos ortus, sic et efficaciam. Medici terreni longam per experientiam, surculorum didicerunt vires, et similium quae permutant qualitates humanorum corporum. Nullus tamen in hac arte sic probatus exstitit, qui non essent ad curandum aliae difficiles, aliaeque passionum prorsus incurabiles. Hoc testatur ille vir Hippocrates qui fuit hoc de coelo sublimatus vir Aesculapius, quibus nemo ventilatur major esse medicus. At supernae medicinae Christus auctor emicat, qui curare sola potest jussione morbidos, et ad vitam de sepulcro revocare mortuos ..." The excerpt given herewith is a portion of the exhortation by means of which an aged priest is represented as having converted Pantaleon. Mention is also made of the imperial physician, Euphrosinus, and of the works of Hippocrates and Esculapius which Pantaleon had studied. The story ends with Pantaleon's conversion on discovering that he could bring to life, by divine aid, a boy who had died from the bite of a poisonous serpent.

[258] Ep. ix (*P. L.,* CXLI). "Crede, pater, nullam me compositionem unguenti laborasse postquam ad ordinem episcopalem accessi, quod tamen pauxillum ex dono cuiusdam medici supererat, mihi fraudans tibi largior. Rogo sospitatis auctore Christo ut tibi illud faciat salutare."

[259] Ep. iv. "Vestrae sospitati amice gratulantes, valetudini quoque vestri fidelis et amici Ebali, si divina benignitas allubescat, quanta novimus ope subvenire paravimus, mittendo Galieni po-

tiones III et totidem theriacae diatesseron; quae quid valeant et modus acceptionis vel servationis earum, in vestris antidotariis facile reperitur. Vulgaginem etiam petitam vobis mittimus, quamvis aetatem vestram tali jam vomitu fatigari non suademus, sed eo potius si opus sit allevari, qui frequenter et sine periculo fieri possit oximelle et raphanis vel certe, quod seniori magis conducibile est, morantem alvum laxativis pillulis incitari. De quibus ultro vobis fere nonaginta oblatis, caetera bona nostra vestra putate. Valete."

[260] See above, notes 43, 44, 144, 187, 189 for descriptions of mss. containing such material. At Chartres, for instance, there are the following mss. from the early centuries, containing materials that were either excerpted from antidotaries such as Fulbert mentioned, or that went into the compilation of such books: ms. 62, from the tenth century, contains (among other medical material) an alphabetical list of simple herbal remedies (f. 54 ff.); ms. 70 (ninth century), f. 126, remedy ad apostema; ms. 102 (tenth century), f. 88, ad cauculos; ms. 74 (tenth century), f. 1 (miscellaneous prescriptions); ms. 53 (eleventh century entry in a ninth century ms.), f. 88, contra migraneam; ms. 193 (eleventh century), f. 187. Chartres has many mss. from the later centuries (twelfth, thirteenth, and fourteenth) in which there are prescriptions, etc.; mss. 223, 284, 398, and 417 contain extended handbooks of remedies. For similar mss. in other French libraries, see P. Pansier, *loc. cit.,* p. 37, under " receptaria."

[261] See H. Sigerist, *Studien und Texte,* and Joerimann, *op. cit.,* for the texts of early medieval *antidotaria* and *receptaria.*

[262] All of the medicaments mentioned by Fulbert are to be found in the texts published by Sigerist and Joerimann (see preceeding note).

[263] Ep. cxviii (*P. L., CXLI*). " Potionem Iera, quam dominus praesul tibi mittit, sumes cum aqua calida ante crepusculum diei. Nocte qua debes eam accipere, non coenabis; et ipso nocte positam potionem in vasculo in quo distemperanda est, asperges salis gemma, vel si haec non adest, delicato sale ad pensum unius scripuli. Accepta potione sedeas ante focum absque ullo tumultu,

cavens tibi penitus a frigore; et si paulum cubueris, non nocebit; nolo tamen ut dormias. Cum primum senties moveri tibi ventrem, deambula pedetentim et sic ad secessum vade. Si propter solutionem tandem ceperit te sitis, nequaquam bibes, nisi paululum aceti cum aqua calida misti, propter stomachum diluendum seu relevandum; quod etiam non urgente siti facere poteris, solutione propemodum vocante. Prandere differes quousque senties catarticum nihil amplius operari velle. Cum sederis ad mensam, vide ne quid nimis, neque manduces aliquid stipticum vel plus aequo salsum. Plura de observationis modo notarem, nisi pauca sufficerent sapienti. Hoc tamen scribere me jubet nescia simulare charitas, ut talem potionis huius sentias effectum, quatenus semper incolumis preserveres. Vale." It is interesting to notice the similarity of treatment in a prescription given by Cato, *De Re Rustica,* ch. clvi; and one (from the ninth century) which appears in Cockayne, *Leechdoms* . . . II, 291. As in Fulbert's prescription, after drinking the potion, the patient was advised to remain quiet until his bowels moved, and then to be very careful about his diet.

[264] *De Sancto Cerauno* (*P. L.,* CXLI).

" Prandia lauta modum turbant plerumque dietae;
Indulges stomacho, mentem male crapula vexat;
Si parcas epulis, sequitur detractio vel laus.
Ut medium teneas labor est, et valde cavendum,
Ne tibi tristitiam pariat, sicut suus est mos.
Si possis igitur, prorsus haec prandia vita,
At si non liceat, hilaris cautusque recumbe,
Et liba cuncta parum, tua quae tibi regula dictat;
Nec summam nimiam conjectent multa minuta."

[265] Adelman of Liége, one of the pupils of Fulbert, wrote a sort of directory, in verse, concerning his fellow students. Concerning Hildegaire he said . . . " Ypocratis artem jungens Socratis sermonibus, Nec minus Pytagoras indulgebat fidebus." Clerval, *op. cit.,* p. 59 ff., publishes the entire poem with a variant text, from a Copenhagen ms. (Bibl. Reg. Gl. Kgl., 1905).

[266] Drogo of Tours, in a letter to Berengar, wrote: " . . . ad

hoc quis non miretur tam in arte medendi qua ipsis, qui se medicos profitentur, premines, excellentiam." H. Sudendorf, *Berengarius Turonensis* (Hamburg, 1850), p. 200.

[267] Ordericus Vitalis, *Historia Ecclesiastica*, V, 18 (*P. L.,* CLXXXVIII); "medicinae artis erat peritissimus."

[268] L. Merlet et Lépinois, *Cartulaire de Notre Dame de Chartres* (Chartres, 1862 ff.), III, 24, indicates that Ralph was a canon of the cathedral chapter. As has been shown by E. Wickersheimer (*op. cit.,* II, 684-5), certain phases of Ralph's career have been grossly exaggerated; notably by Dubreuil-Chambardel, *op. cit.,* 23 ff. Wickersheimer's words, " a romantic biography," are justly applicable to many of the statements found in the works of both Dubreuil-Chambardel and Clerval concerning the medical attainments of certain of their heroes. Wickersheimer's recently published work displays a critical acumen that is an excellent check on the overly optimistic tendencies of many of the other French historians of medicine.

[269] William of Jumièges, *Gesta Normannorum Ducum* (*P. L.,* CXLIX, mentions the early phases of Ralph's career (VII, 10). Ordericus Vitalis, *op. cit.,* III, 5, 11, tells of his Italian journey, and of his later reputation for marvelous cures in northern France.

[270] Richer, *Historia*, II, 59. Although the tale is too long to quote, it contains several points of importance. The Salernitan was the Queen's favorite physician, whereas the King preferred the French bishop. Both were represented as " peritissimus in arte medicinae," but the French bishop had a broad background of education " artibus literarum," whereas the Salernitan, " nulla literarum scientia imbutus," had wide experience in practical matters. In the conflict of wits, the Frenchman, a cleric and physician with a liberal arts education easily triumphs over the Salernitan, a laymen and a narrowly practical physician. Thus, whether truth or legend, the tale indicates the trend of French medicine, and the prejudice of French trained physicians against upstart Italians. The same tendency is noticeable in the story of Ralph's visit to Salerno.

[271] Dubreuil-Chambardel, *op. cit.*, p. 23 ff. and 232-4 gives a detailed account (with some of the original texts) concerning Ralph's later exploits. As indicated above, however (note 268), Dubreuil-Chambardel is inclined to exaggerate the achievements of French physicians.

[272] The signatures appear in the following order: " Guilduinus vicecomes . . . Harduinus vicecomes filius eius, Elisabeth uxor eiusdem, *Johannes medicus, Guiszo medicus,* Girbertus presbyter . . . (etc., including the signatures of the " princeps cocorum vicecomitis," " pincerna comitis," " cellarius," " cocus," and finally " Ericus puer "). The charter is found in Guérard, *Cartulaire de Saint-Père,* I, 160-2; also, along with numerous " pièces justificatives," in Dubreuil-Chambardel, *op. cit.*, p. 231.

[273] There is considerable uncertainty as to the exact facts concerning physicians of the eleventh century named John. During this century, in the region of France there seems to have been dozens of that name. See for instance the index of Dubreuil-Chambardel, *op. cit.*, or Wickersheimer's *Dictionnaire Biographique,* I, 342 ff., which lists well over a hundred " Johns," to say nothing of over fifty pages of physicians with some sort of family name in addition to the surname " John." We cannot, therefore, be certain that the John who served the Count of Anjou was the same John who studied at Chartres. One thing is certain, John of Chartres became a famous physician in northern France, and it was he who served King Henry I of France (see next note). See Wickersheimer, *op. cit.*, II, 488.

[274] Ordericus Vitalis, *op. cit.*, III, 12. " Henricus rex Francorum post multas probitates quibus in regno gloriose viguit, potionem a *Joanne medico Carnotensi,* qui ex eventu Surdus cognominabatur, spe longioris vitae accepit. Sed quia voto suo magis quam praecepto archiatri absecundavit, et aquam, dum veneno rimante interiora nimis angeretur, clam a cubiculario sitiens poposcit, medicoque ignorante, ante purgationem bibit. Proh dolor! in crastinum cum magno multorum moerore obiit." William of Jumièges, *op. cit.*, VII, 28, gives a similar account.

[275] Richer, *Historia,* III, 96. "Post eum ex indigestione Romae laboraret, et intestini squibalas ex melancolico humore pateretur, aloen ad pondus dragmarum quatuor sanitatis avidus sumpsit. Conturbatisque visceribus, diarria iugus prosecuta est. Cuius continuus fluxus, emorroides tumentes procreavit. Quae sanguinem immoderatum effundentes, mortem post dies non plures operatae sunt."

[276] See above, note 274; "Ex eventu Surdus cognominabatur."

[277] Wickersheimer, *op. cit.,* I, 64.

[278] See *ibid.* for the known facts concerning the medical careers of the men mentioned in this paragraph. This work is preferable to those of Clerval, *op. cit.,* and Dubreuil-Chambardel, *op. cit.*

[279] E. g., "Bernardo medico," "Richerius medicus," "Domnus medicus," "Goslenus medicus" (all three quoted by Clerval, *op. cit.,* p. 200, from ,cartularies); "Laurentius medicus de Sancto Dionisio" (Wickersheimer, *op. cit.,* II, 519); "Johannes medicus" (Clerval, *op. cit.,* p. 320; Jean, "apothecarius phisicus"; Guillaume de Villeneuve, "phisicus"; Geoffroi "medicus"; Guillaume de Leves "apothecarius de Carnoto"; André "phisicus"; Olivier, "phisicus"; Thibaud, "cirurgicus"; Pierre du Moi, "cirurgicus"; Pierre de Troyes, "apothecarius," etc. (Clerval, *op. cit.,* p. 370-1; and Wickersheimer, *op. cit.,* under each name).

[280] In all probability the *herborii, pigmentarii,* and various other assistants who performed the menial routine activities of medical practice, were laymen. See above, note 251, and also the excellent account of this aspect of medicine in Dubreuil-Chambardel, *op. cit.,* p. 212 ff.

[281] Guérard, *Cartulaire de Saint-Père de Chartres,* contains names and titles such as the following (from the twelfth century): Gaucelin *minutor,* Gislebert *minutor,* Girardus *rasator* and *rasorius* (see index). For evidence of lay barbers, surgeons, etc., elsewhere, see Dubreuil-Chambardel, *op. cit.,* p. 213 ff.

[282] In the following mss. (from the twelfth, thirteenth, and fourteenth centuries) the following treatises are to be found:

Hippocrates *Aphorisms* in mss. 160, 171, 278, 286; Hippocrates *Prognostics* in mss. 160, 171, 278, 286; Hippocrates *de dieta acutarum* . . . , in mss. 278 and 286; a great variety of Galen's works are found in mss. 284 and 293, and the ars medicina in mss. 286 and 287. Alexander of Tralles *Therapeutica* appears in ms. 342 (this appears to have been copied from the former Chartres ms., now Paris B. N. 9332); Theophilus *liber de urinis* is in mss. 160, 171, 278, 286; Philaretus *liber pulsuum* in mss. 160, 171, 278, 286, and 393; the *ysagoge Johannicii* in mss. 160, 171, 278, and 286; Avicenna *Canon* in mss. 223, 278, and 313; Hebenmesue *de simplicibus* in ms. 398; works attributed to Constantine the African appear in mss. 132, 160, and 393; works of John of Saint Amand, in mss. 223 and 398; Gentil de Fulgineo, in mss. 403 and 381 (fifteenth century ms.); Bernard de Gordonio in mss. 224 and 393; Dino de Garbo in ms. 403; Aegidius de Corbel's verses *de pulsibus et urinis*, in ms. 393; and various other works in mss. 307, 393, 398, 403, 425, 555, and 1029. There are a few medical mss. from the fifteenth and sixteenth centuries which I have not listed. G. Cormer, *Anatomical Texts of the Earlier Middle Ages* (Washington, 1927), contains valuable material concerning an uncatalogued text from ms. 284.

[283] Mss. 224, 278, 293, and 417 were donated by Pierre Bechebien. Mss. 286 and 313 were given by " Magister Laurencius de Tumesnil," a member of the cathedral chapter; ms. 284, by " Magister Nicolaus de Mola Medici "; and ms. 223 by " Theobaldus de Pertouville," another member of the cathedral chapter.

[284] Ms. 1036, "Apothecarius moralis Monasterii Sancti Petri Carnotensis "; f. 3 contains the frontispiece miniature (see plate IX); f. 54-60 comprises a *liber de sanitate conservandi,* of medical remedies. B. N. ms. 9332 (eighth century) has a miniature which shows the same tendency of paralleling medical and religious activities (see plate III).

PLATES

PLATE I

Early in the ninth century a plan was drawn up for the rebuilding
and expansion of the monastic buildings. The above plan represents
the section that was to be built at one corner of the monastic enclosure for the care of the sick monks. Evidently they were segregated from the rest of the community; note the separate church for
the sick. There were separate quarters elsewhere for sick novices
and for visitors and the poor. Note the special quarters for those
who were seriously ill, for the doctors, and for the chief physician
(*medici ipsius*). See note 98, and p. 54 f.

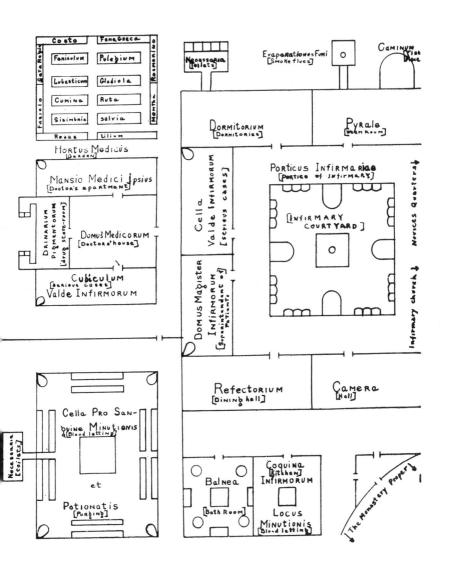

215

PLATE II

Chartres ms. 62 folio 14 (tenth century)

This folio contains the last six entries in the table of contents and the opening lines of the prologue of the *Aurelius,* a popular medieval handbook of remedies arranged according to diseases "from head to foot." This manuscript was probably in use at Chartres at the time of Fulbert, Heribrand, and Richer. Richer seems to have quoted from it in his *Historia.* (see above p. 129 f.).

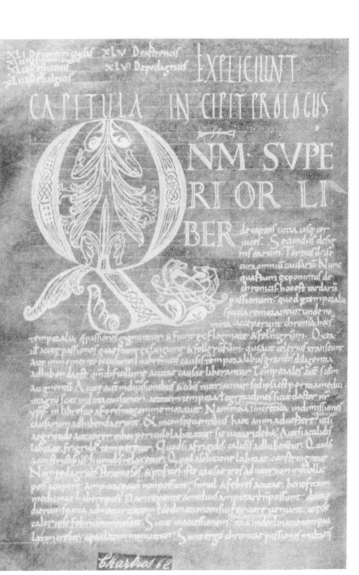

EXPLICIUNT
CAPITULA INCIPIT PROLOGUS

QNM· SVPE
RIOR LI
BER

217

PLATE III

A Classical Medical Treatise From Chartres or Fleury

Paris B. N. lat. ms. 9332 folio 140 (eighth century)

This is the frontispiece of the *Therapeutica* of Alexander of Tralles. The manuscript, which was brought to Paris from Chartres in the eighteenth century, is thought by some scholars to have originated at Fleury (see notes 213, 218). It is the earliest extant example of the Latin translations of Alexander's famous treatise which was written in Greek in the fourth century and translated into Latin about two centuries later in or near Ravenna. The seated figure is Alexander. The title reads " Alexander Sapiens Medicus exposuit unum libellum artis medicinae." The section to the right, containing a cross and scriptural words, illustrates the medieval tendency to combine " earthly medicine " with " heavenly healing." (see plate IX).

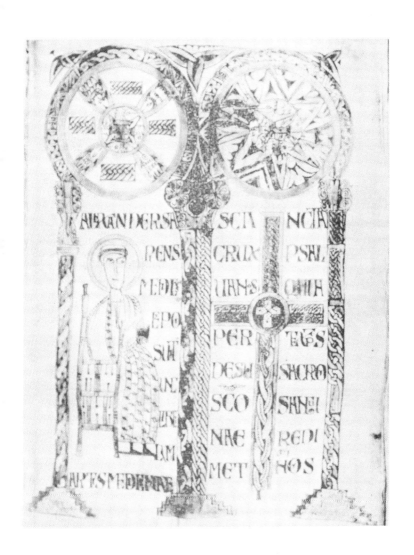

ALEXANDER SA
PENS
MEDIT
EPO
SUI
ANI
MVM
CARPES MEDICINAE

SCIA NCTA
CRUX PSAL
LIANS OMLH
PER TEES
DESI SACRO
SCO SANCT
NAE REDI
MET HOS

219

PLATE IV

A STRAY MEDICAL LETTER FROM CHARTRES OR FLEURY

Paris B. N. lat. ms. 9332 folio 251 (eighth century)

This *Epistula Uulter,* a curious letter concerning diseases and remedies, was inserted in the manuscript on a blank sheet at the end of book I of the *Materia Medica* of Dioscorides. Often brief medical treatises such as this were written on spare pages of manuscripts. This letter is similar in form to the many brief, general treatises of the early middle ages which were attributed to famous classical physicians such as Hippocrates and Galen. See note 213.

PLATE V

The Oldest Latin Manuscript of Oribasius

Paris B. N. lat. ms. 10233 folio 134 (sixth-eighth century)

This is a folio from Oribasius' *Synopsis,* a Graeco-Latin treatise which was translated into Latin during the fifth or sixth century at Ravenna. Copies doubtless circulated throughout France during the pre-Carolingian period for there are three Oribasius manuscripts from this period in French libraries today. The folio shown above is in uncial script, badly faded. The manuscript was formerly at Chartres, and perhaps came originally from Fleury (see notes 211-12).

PLATE VI

A MEDICAL PRESCRIPTION FROM FLEURY

Paris B. N. lat. ms. 6400 B folio 86 (tenth-eleventh century)

Although Fleury was a famous educational center in the early middle ages, and possessed many manuscripts, they have been scattered far and wide during modern times (see note 223). This folio is from one of the few known medical manuscripts of Fleury; the Fleury library marks are to be found on several of the folios. Prescriptions such as the one shown above, concerning *Oleum Savininum,* were very common. Most of them came originally from classical handbooks (those of Hippocrates, Galen, Pliny, etc.). Note the reference to Galen's treatise *ad Glauconem* on line 18.

Oleum saminū eū facere adeuenī mitissimū

corē prū de electam ʒ ℈ oleū libras ...
Oleū ... ʒ aut ... remollar uide coques.
donec unū sicerur · Abigne iacet & proiec
erbam remaslam · Oleum aūt in ampulla
mitris & altis diseminā met ʒ · Conuenit ad
articulo cum dolore · Subuincm ... fiet
opus est · est enī calidū nimis Adiaforeticas
& calide nacur ... inflacof · Ol saminū ad
experis dolore · emendanda & aduersi inon
collendū of lib .iii. ede re mel libec sapē
moriae sucū lib i sarpullisiciū lib i pule
sucū lib i saune sucū lib i aceri lib i liecoma
coques in aceto & molla usq̃ sucus & acerū
consomar ... & colas & aliis puluerem debasi
laur i mirrā & agitas forbiter & sic repones
in uase utetis cum opus fuerit ·

Adienus ad glauconem Oleū saluninum
omnium tenuissimē ... & pene&rabilis
cui uir ture curau te presente inferiorem
creatis cui cossa cota eu neruis & musculis
scirosin quasi lapis fuerat inmobilis facta
& herisipilaca male · & contra ue curau eu ...
curacioni egomor enim aduertii debere me
adhibere medicamina subtile & tenui cuiʃ...
te ... ture que & soluere ualeant & dolo
malro & calido oleo saunino diutissime fo
...talis · & nere frigeraran post fomentacionē
deter ... ebam · & sic diaforetics ... eram certas

225

PLATE VII

MEDICAL SHORTHAND FROM RHEIMS

Paris B. N. lat. ms. 8780 folio 39 (ninth century)

From Rheims originally came this manuscript of Tironian notes (i. e., shorthand), which were much used in the early centuries. There are two pages of medical terms and their corresponding symbols, such as is shown above. Most of the words are the names of diseases; for instance, ulcer, fever, etc. (see note 232).

PLATE VIII

A Medical Treatise in Verse From Rheims

Paris B. N. lat. ms. 9347 folio 57 (ninth century)

In Gerbert's day Rheims had many medical manuscripts, but, like those of Fleury, they were dispersed. Today only one small excerpt is in existence; a nine page section containing the beginning and end of the poetical *Liber Medicinalis* of Quintus Serenus Sammonicus. Above is shown the last section, containing the *Explicit Lib. Medicinalis Quinti Sereni.* See p. 120 f.

PLATE IX

Chartres ms. 1036, folio 3 (fourteenth century)

The high rank given to medicine by the monastic mind is indicated by the frequent association of medical with religious activities
in medieval writings. There are frequent references to " earthly and
celestial " medicine, and occasionally one finds illustrations such as
this, comparing medical treatment with spiritual healing (see also
plate III). The panels at the right represent religious sacraments;
those at the left, medical activities; urine analysis in a physician's
office (upper), and an apothecary and his assistant compounding
drugs (lower). The manuscript in which the illustration appears
bears the appropriate title, *Apothecarius Moralis*; it was a general
compendium of information, both religious and secular. (see note
284).

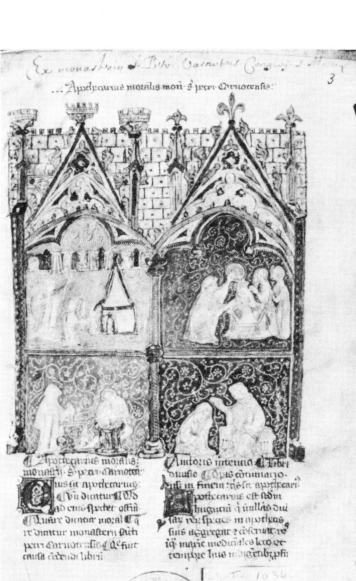

INDEX

A

Abascantus of Lyons, 176
abdomen, 43, 129, see belly
Abelard, 12
Accius Justus, 98, 179, 189, 191
aconite, 38
acute diseases, 83
adder, bite of, 30, see snake, bite of
Adelman of Liége, 207
Adrianus, 167
Aegidius of Corbeil, 211
ages of man, 97, 190
Agricola of Chalons, 178
Agriculture, by Cato, 33
agridium, 63
Aix-la-Chapelle, 90 f., 192 ff.
Alaric, 10, 16
Alcuin, 40, 82, 85 ff., 186 f.
Alexander of Tralles, 48, 77, 98, 111 f., 189, 196, 211, 218 f.
Alexandria, 16
Alfred (the Great), 8
alms house, 102, see guest house, hospice, *xenodochia*
aloes, 143
alphabetical treatises, 146, 206, see glossary, synonyms
Amatus of Chartres, 110
America, colonial medicine, 33, 172
amputation, 41, 203
amulet, 29
anatomy, 83, 145
Angers, 149

Anglo-Saxon medicine, 52, 54, 158, 166, 168, see England
Anjou, 143
Ansbert of Rouen, 178
antebalumina (*antiballomena*), 167, 181, 191
Anthimus of Constantinople, 42 ff., 70, 77, 90, 162
antidotaria, 31, 36, 135 f., 167, 180, 189 ff., 206
antidote, 32, 52, 63, 67, 78, 88, 136 f., 167, 190, 201
antidote philanthropos, 116
Antiochus, King, 189 f.
anus, 130
Aphorisms, of Hippocrates, 98, 122, 125 f., 190
Apollo, 16, 21, 188
Apollonius, 191
apoplexy, 190
apostema, 117
apothecarius, apothecary, 40, 131, 145 f., 210, 230 f.
Apothecarius Moralis, 146, 211, 230
Apuleius, 32
Apuleius Plato, 180
Aquileia, 182
Arabic medicine, 94, 146, 150
archiater, 18, 44, 47 ff., 69 ff., 143, 174, see royal physician
Aristotle, 10
arithmetic and medicine, 96
Arles, 73 f., 176, 193
arm, 33
Armentarius, 67

heart, 64, 189
heartburn, 129
Heliodorus, 181, 189 f.
hemorrhage, 46, 62
hemorrhoids, 130, 144, 191
Henry I of France, 143
herbarii, 131, 210
herbs, 22-38, 51-55, 63, 78,
    86 ff., 103, 127, 134, 167 ff.,
    172, 177, 180, 184, 189, 191,
    206, 210, see simples
Heribrand of Chartres, 121 ff.,
    126 ff., 132 f., 216
hermeneumata, 78, 189, 196
hermit, 63, 71
Hermogenis, 167
hernia, 73
hernia bandages, 176
hiera potion, 137 ff.
Hildegaire, 137, 139
Hippocrates, 44, 51 ff., 77 f., 86,
    97 f., 122 ff., 134, 139, 146,
    167, 180 f., 184, 189 ff., 202,
    205, 211
History, by Richer, 128 ff.
History of the Franks, by
    Gregory of Tours, 62
holy water, 17, 30
horehound, 38
Hortulus of Walafrid Strabo,
    36, 41, 53, 169
hospice, 71, 74 ff., 99, 101 ff.,
    170, 177, 179, 193 ff., see
    guest house, *xenodochia*
hospital, 15, 55, 74, 76, 99 ff.,
    149, 170, 177, 179, 192 f.,
    see infirmary
hospitalia Scotorum, 179, 192
Hôtel Dieu, Paris, 179, 192

Huguenots, and Fleury library,
    113, 199
humanist, 124
humors, 43, 82 f., 97, 130,
    189 f.
Hungarians, 107
hyssop, 63, 183

I

ileum, 130
impotency, 32
incantations, 22 ff., 28 ff., 87,
    191
infant, 41
infirmarius, 74
infirmary, 40, 54 f., 74 ff., 79,
    99, 151, 177, 191, 199, 214 f.,
    see hospital
infirmities, 182
inguen, 130
insane, 64
insomnia, 190
interrogationes, 97
intestines, 34, 129 f.
intoxication, 138
Irish, 9, 54, 187, see Scots
Isaac the Jew, 187
Isidore of Seville, 20, 82, 95
Iso of St. Gall, 38
Italian medicine, 1, 13, 25, 36,
    42, 47 ff., 50, 55, 60, 69, 78,
    81, 85 f., 104, 111, 114, 141,
    150, 181, 184, 187, 195, 200
Ivo of Chartres, 145

J

Jews, 36, 68, 70, 94, 170, 187
John the physician of Chartres,
    142 ff., 209

240

Martyrs, The Glories of, 62
Masona of Merida, 170
materia medica, 77 f., 111, 169, 197, 202
mathematics, 116
Maurus, Rabanus, 26 f., 82 f., 88, 94 f., 131, 146
measures, see weights and measures
meat, 43, 89
Meaux, council of, 192
medicaments, 66, 84, 87, 94, 127, 183, see compounds, drugs, pharmacy, prescriptions, simples
Medicina, de, of Celsus, 118
medicus, 40, 45, 69 ff., 131, 134, 145, 170, 191, 210, 214 f., 218, see doctor, physician.
melancholia, 83
melon seed, 34
members, four, 190
memory, remedy for improving, 32
mercurial remedies, 35
Merida, Spain, 41, 170
Merovingian medicine, 24, 60 ff., 74, 103 ff., 144, 171, 177
Mesue's *de simplicibus,* 211
metals, 35, 128
Methodist (medical school), 124
midwife, 22, 31, 72
milk, 43
Minerva, 16
minutor, (bloodletter), 145, 210, 215
miraculous healing, 17 ff., 23 ff., 30, 45, 61 ff., 71, 82, 134,

156 f., 172, 205, see relics, saints
missi dominici, 101
Moerland, H., 165
Molinier, A., 195
monthly observations, 53, 191
Monte Cassino, 18, 36, 52, 54, 93
Monte Cassino, manuscripts of, 52 f., 167
Moorish Spain, 94
Moors, 107
Morbis, de, of Alexander of Tralles, 98
morbus regius, 196 f.
Morigund, 71
mouth, 24, 35 f., 63
mules, surgery of, 65
municipal physicians, 48 f., 72 f.
music and medicine, 96
mussels, 33

N

ŋard, 135 f.
nasal hemorrhage, 46
Natural History, see Pliny
nausea, 129
navel, 129
Nepotianus, 190
Neuburger, M., 165
Nicolaus de Mola, 211
Nivelles, hospice at, 179
Normandy, 140, 144
Norse, 8, 107, 113, 154
Notker of St. Gall, 46
nursing, 15, 72, 76, 80, 95, 177
nutmeg, 34

Walsh, Dr. J., 19
water, 37, 138, 143, 191
weights and measures, 53, 78, 138, 167, 180, 188 ff., 196
Wickersheimer, Dr. E., 208 f.
Williams, Roger, 60
William of Conches, 145
William the Conqueror, 144
winds, the four, 190
wine, 37, 86, 89, 138, 186, 191, 203
witch, 1, 22
women, 71 f., see gynecology
wound, 34, 37, 41 f., 48, 78, 146, 175, 182

X

xenodochia, 74, 100, 170, 177 ff., 193 f., see guest house, hospice

Y

Young, Brigham, 60
ΤΠΑΤΙΚΟΝ, 117
ypocundria, 130
Ysagoge, 97, 190, 211

Z

Zilboorg, Dr. G., 1 f.

JOHNS HOPKINS UNIVERSITY PRESS REPRINTS

An Arno Press Collection

Agard, Walter Raymond. **The Greek Tradition in Sculpture.** 1930

Allen, Don Cameron. **Doubt's Boundless Sea: Skepticism and Faith in the Renaissance.** 1964

Bailey, Thomas A. **The Policy of the United States Toward the Neutrals, 1917-1918.** 1942

Barton, John. **Observations on the Circumstances Which Influence the Condition of the Labouring Classes of Society.** 1934

Beall, Otho T. and Richard H. Shryock. **Cotton Mather: First Significant Figure in American Medicine.** 1954

Beardsley, Grace Hadley. **The Negro in Greek and Roman Civilization.** 1929

Bloomfield, Maurice and Richard Garbe, eds. **The Kashmirian Atharva-Veda.** 1901

Bloomfield, Maurice. **The Life and Stories of the Jaina Savior Parcvanatha.** 1919

Boas, George. **Wingless Pegasus: A Handbook for Critics.** 1950

Carr, Edward Hallett. **German-Soviet Relations Between the Two World Wars, 1919-1939.** 1951

German-Soviet Relations Between the Two World Wars, 1919-1939. 1951

Castiglioni, Arturo. **The Renaissance of Medicine in Italy.** 1934

Chinard, Gilbert, ed. **The Correspondence of Jefferson and Du Pont De Nemours.** 1931

Chinard, Gilbert, ed. **Un Français En Virginie: Voyages d'un François Exilé pour la Réligion avec une Déscription de la Virgine & Marilan dans L'Amérique.** 1932

Chinard, Gilbert, ed. **Houdon in America.** 1930

Chinard, Gilbert, ed. **The Letters of Lafayette and Jefferson.** 1929

Chinard, Gilbert, ed. **Souvenirs D'Édouard De Mondésir.** 1942

Chinard, Gilbert, ed. **The Treaties of 1778 and Allied Documents.** 1928

Chinard, Gilbert, ed. **La Vie Americaine De Guillaume Merle D'Aubigné.** 1935

Chinard, Gilbert, ed. **Voyage dans L'Intérieur des Etats-Unis et au Canada par Le Comte de Colbert Maulevrier.** 1935

Chinard, Gilbert, ed. **Le Voyage de Lapérouse sur les Côtes de L'Alaska et de la Californie.** 1937

Daugherty, William E. **A Psychological Warfare Casebook.** 1958

Drazin, Nathan. **History of Jewish Education from 515 B.C.E. to 220 C.E.** 1940

Dyer, Murray. **The Weapon on the Wall: Rethinking Psychological Warfare.** 1959

French, John C. **A History of the University Founded by Johns Hopkins.** 1946

Galt, John. **The Gathering of the West.** 1939

Gildersleeve, Basil. **The Creed of the Old South, 1865-1915.** 1915

Goodnow, Frank J. **China: An Analysis.** 1926

Hardy, Thomas. **An Indiscretion in the Life of an Heiress.** 1935

Jones, W.H.S. **Philosophy and Medicine in Ancient Greece.** 1946

Korson, George. **Black Rock: Mining Folklore of the Pennsylvania Dutch.** 1960

Korson, George, ed. **Pennsylvania Songs and Legends.** 1949

Lane, Frederic Chapin. **Venetian Ships and Shipbuilders of the Renaissance.** 1934

Langer, Susanne K. **Philosophical Sketches.** 1962

Langer, Susanne K., ed. **Reflections on Art.** 1958

Lumiansky, R.M., ed. **Malory's Originality: A Critical Study of Le Morte Darthur.** 1964

MacKinney, Loren C. **Early Medieval Medicine with Special Reference to France and Chartres.** 1937

Martin-Clarke, D. Elizabeth. **Culture in Early Anglo Saxon England.** 1947

Miller, Genevieve, ed. **Bibliography of the History of Medicine of the United States and Canada, 1939-1960.** 1964

Newsholme, Arthur. **Public Health and Insurance: American Addresses.** 1920

Oliphant, Herman and Theodore S. Hope, Jr. **A Study of Day Calendars.** 1932

Painter, Sidney. **The Reign of King John.** 1949

Qubain, Fahim I. **Education and Science in the Arab World.** 1966

Remer, C.F. **A Study of Chinese Boycotts.** 1933

Ricardo, David. **Letters of John Ramsay McCulloch to David Ricardo** *and* **Three Letters on the Price of Gold,** Two vols. in one. 1931/1903

Ricardo, David. **Minor Papers on the Currency Question, 1809-1823.** 1932

Semmes, Raphael. **Captains and Mariners of Early Maryland.** 1937

Shanks, Lewis Piaget. **Flaubert's Youth, 1821-1845.** 1927

Sigerist, Henry E. **Four Treatises of Theophrastus Von Hohenheim Called Paracelsus.** 1941

Simmons, James Stevens, et al. **Malaria in Panama.** 1939

Simonds, Frank H. **American Foreign Policy in the Post-War Years.** 1935

Spector, Benjamin, ed. **Noah Webster: Letters on Yellow Fever Addressed to Dr. William Currie.** 1947

Suhr, Elmer G. **Sculptured Portraits of Greek Statesmen.** 1931

Suhr, Elmer G. **Two Currents in the Thought Stream of Europe.** 1942

Tabak, Israel. **Judaic Lore in Heine.** 1948

Turnbull, Grace H., ed. **Tongues of Fire: A Bible of Sacred Scriptures of the Pagan World.** 1941

Willoughby, Westel W. **Japan's Case Examined.** 1940

Young, C. Walter. **The International Legal Status of the Kwantung Leased Territory.** 1931

Young, C. Walter. **Japanese Jurisdiction in the South Manchuria Railway Areas.** 1931

Young, C. Walter. **Japan's Special Position in Manchuria.** 1931

Zeeland, Paul van. **A View of Europe, 1932.** 1933

Zimmer, Henry R. **Hindu Medicine.** 1948